Caring for People with Multiple Disabilities

An Interdisciplinary Guide for Caregivers

by

Cindy French, O.T.R.

Robin Tapp González, M.A., CCC-SLP

Jan Tronson-Simpson, R.P.T.

Illustrations drawn under contract
by Cathie Lowmiller

Therapy Skill Builders™ ®
a division of
The Psychological Corporation

555 Academic Court
San Antonio, Texas 78204-2498
1-800-228-0752

WD

Reproducing Pages from This Book

Several of the pages in this book may be reproduced for instructional or administrative use (not for resale). To protect your book, make a photocopy of each reproducible page. Then, use that copy as a master for photocopying or other types of reproduction.

About the Authors

Cindy French, O.T.R., received the B.S. degree in occupational therapy from the University of Kansas and is certified in pediatric NDT treatment. Currently in private practice in the Denver area, Ms. French consults for several group homes for children and adults with developmental disabilities and for several local preschools. Although her current professional emphasis is on pediatric treatment, she has worked in a variety of settings with clients of all ages.

Robin Tapp González, M.A., CCC-SLP, received the M.A. degree in speech and language pathology from the University of Denver and is certified in pediatric NDT treatment. She is in private practice, serving primarily pediatric clients. As a consulting speech-language pathologist to several group homes for school-aged children with multiple handicaps, she provides ongoing inservice training to professional and paraprofessional staff members. Ms. González also is employed by a state-run residential, educational, and vocational training center for people with developmental disabilities.

Jan Tronson-Simpson, R.P.T., received the B.S. degree in physical therapy from the University of Colorado and is certified in pediatric NDT treatment. Ms. Tronson-Simpson has been in private practice, specializing in infants and children who have developmental disabilities and neurological impairments. She consulted for several group homes for children and adults with developmental disabilities. Her previous position was as pediatric specialist at Lutheran Medical Center, where she was part of a team that developed a pediatric program to follow up and treat high-risk infants. She has recently relocated to Saudi Arabia, where she has been providing NDT treatment to Saudi infants, children, and young adults at Dhahran Health Center.

Contents

Preface vii

1. Introduction and Historical Perspective 1

2. Muscle Tone and Handling Techniques............................... 7

3. Range of Motion 19

4. Influence of Abnormal Reflexes.. 41

5. Sensory Impairments 47

6. Positioning 53

7. Feeding and Oral-Motor Concerns 63

8. Dental Hygiene 97

9. Bathing and Dressing... 101

10. Communication 107

11. Switch Mechanisms 115

12. Fine Motor Guidelines... 121

13. Gross Motor Guidelines 125

14. Play and Recreation... 129

Glossary of Therapy Terms 135

Appendix: Equipment Sources... 139

Bibliography 145

Preface

We are a team of consulting therapists who represent the disciplines of physical, occupational, and speech-language therapies. Through providing services to individuals with physical and mental disabilities in group-home settings, we identified a need for a reference guide to be used by caregivers. Caregivers can make a marked difference in a client's life, particularly if they are well informed and can actively participate in therapeutic intervention. This manual has been designed, therefore, to give caretakers an understanding of therapeutic principles and their application. The direct-care staff can then apply this information to specific programs or activities of daily living with their clients. We hope this manual will be of interest to a variety of professionals and paraprofessionals:

- Direct-care staff working with individuals who have multiple handicaps
- Professional consultants who wish to have a reference for inservice presentations
- Family members of individuals with multiple disabilities who are living at home
- Administrators within alternative-care settings who want orientation information for new employees

This information is applicable to individuals aged five through adult. For accessibility, we have made every effort to limit the use of terminology specific to our disciplines and to explain terms that may be unfamiliar. We feel this publication is a cost-effective and time-efficient means of presenting pertinent information.

In each chapter, the area of concern will be described or defined, followed by examples of how related therapeutic principles can be applied in clients' daily lives. Chapters 2 through 6 present information about the conditions a person with developmental disabilities may have and address therapeutic methods of intervention. Chapters 7 through 11 emphasize daily-care and socialization issues. Information regarding fine and gross motor skills is covered in chapters 12 and 13. The final chapter is devoted to play and leisure skills and is followed by a glossary of terms used in the manual and a list of sources for specialized equipment. The principles described are general and apply to a variety of disabilities and age ranges. Treatment suggestions are practical and goal-directed. Reproducibles are included to assist with inservices and daily programming.

1

Introduction and Historical Perspective

Until the 1950s, people with psychiatric impairments, mental retardation, or physical disabilities were typically segregated from society and housed in institutions. As a result of changes in societal attitudes and federal laws, the 1960s and 1970s saw a movement away from institution-based care toward community-based residential care. Many people who would have been institutionalized in the past now live in new care settings such as group homes or alternative community residences. These individuals, due to their limited physical or mental abilities, usually need constant services and assistance to function within the community.

A *community-based residence* is simply a homelike setting that provides services twenty-four hours a day to a small group of persons with disabilities. Several options for community-based residences are currently available, depending on your state and the agencies that provide services in your area. Examples include foster family care, community residences or group homes, shared apartments, or apartments with varying degrees of supervision. In some areas, state schools, developmental centers, or skilled nursing facilities containing more than forty persons with developmental disabilities continue to operate. Regardless of where they live, clients today participate in many outside services—vocational, educational, habilitative, or recreational—that help them integrate into the community.

Since the 1970s, the caregiving approach in the public sector has shifted from a custodial, maintenance model to an active treatment, community-based model. *Active treatment* is a philosophy that encourages individuals to participate in formal and informal programming throughout the day, rather than being passively moved through activities of daily living by a staff member. *Formal programming* refers to structured therapy activities in which the resident participates with staff supervision or assistance. These structured therapy activities are usually specified in the person's *Individual Habilitation Plan* (IHP), with the goal of making the individual more independent in one or more areas of life. Less structured, socially or therapeutically based activities are referred to as *informal programming* within active treatment. These activities can be more community-based and may not have to be documented as rigorously.

Since the 1970s, various definitions have been developed for the term *developmental disabilities*. One of the most widely accepted definitions is from PL 95-602, the Rehabilitation Comprehensive Services and Developmental Disabilities Amendment of 1978 to the Developmentally Disabled Assistance and Bill of Rights Act. This definition states:

> The term 'developmental disability' means a severe, chronic disability of a person which:
>
> (A) is attributable to a mental or physical impairment or combination of mental and physical impairments;
>
> (B) is manifested before the person reaches age 22;
>
> (C) is likely to continue indefinitely;
>
> (D) results in substantial limitations in three or more of the following areas of major life activity: (i) self-care, (ii) receptive and expressive language, (iii) learning, (iv) mobility, (v) self-direction, (vi) capacity for independent living, and (vii) economic self-sufficiency; and
>
> (E) reflects the person's need for a combination and sequence of special, interdisciplinary or generic care, treatment or other services which are of lifelong or extended duration and are individually planned and coordinated.

Developmental delay and developmental disability are general terms that imply the presence of multiple handicaps or delays in several areas of development. Two people with the same diagnosis may have extremely different functional abilities, strengths, and needs. In many cases, people with developmental delays are diagnosed with autism, cerebral palsy, epilepsy, mental retardation, or other neurological or systemic impairments. These terms should be differentiated from *slow growth* or *slow learning* because the physical consequences of a developmental disability generally worsen with increased growth and development, due to the effects of abnormal neurological influences and muscle-tone fluctuations. An individual with multiple disabilities may show severe neurological, medical, and orthopedic (skeletal) conditions that involve the entire body. It is important to remember, however, that each individual with a developmental disability is unique, just as any two "normal" people are different. Some of the general characteristics of the developmentally disabled population may include the following:

1. The person may need assistance to move or may be essentially unable to move independently.

2. If the person can move independently, movements are often abnormal or nonpurposeful.

3. Communication is typically difficult, and many persons are nonverbal.

4. The person may show self-abusive or aggressive behaviors.

5. Frequent medical problems include chronic respiratory infections or aspiration (inhaling secretions, food, or liquid into the lungs).

6. The person may have difficulty eating due to problems with sucking, swallowing, or chewing. Concomitant digestive problems may cause malnutrition and constipation.

7. Bowel or urinary problems are common, as is incontinence. Some clients do not have urinary control and must wear diapers.

8. Seizure activity and side effects of seizure-controlling medications may influence the person's level of functioning.

9. Hearing and visual problems are frequently present, either because of physical impairments or from unknown causes.

10. Individuals typically have limited cognitive skills, often with IQs ranging from 0 to 30.

Because of this multiplicity of problems—poor communication, limited thinking skills, lack of independent physical movement and self-care abilities, ongoing medical conditions, and socially inappropriate behaviors—individuals with developmental disabilities require supervision to ensure a healthy and safe environment. Appropriate management in all areas of development can prevent further deterioration of the person's skills and improve the quality of the individual's life.

The treatment team or staff that works together to assist the client with developmental disabilities can include many specialists: physical therapists, occupational therapists, speech-language pathologists, audiologists, psychologists, dieticians/nutritionists, nurses, physicians, dentists, orthotists/prosthetists, and others. In addition, and just as important, there is the direct-care staff and the people who manage them, whether house managers or administrators. Through a combined effort of all these people, the client can achieve the highest possible level of functioning. Understanding the role of each specialist on the interdisciplinary team can help you direct your questions and concerns to the correct therapist.

The *physical therapist* generally concentrates on the client's overall functional ability, looking particularly at control and purpose of movement. This therapist tests muscle tone, joint range of motion, muscle strength, movement patterns (normal and abnormal), and posture. Reflexes, motor development, coordination, balance, and movement planning skills are also evaluated. After assessing the client, the physical therapist then designs a treatment program. The physical therapist can answer questions about bracing for the trunk and legs and about positioning or assisting with movement.

The focus of *occupational therapy* is to develop or improve functional skills, including play, self-care skills, and prevocational or vocational training, depending on the age and goals of the client. The occupational therapist looks at muscle tone and strength, joint range of motion, movement patterns, and reflexes, particularly when they affect fine motor skills. *Fine motor skills* are tasks or movements requiring use of the hands, arms, and shoulders, and movements of the mouth and jaw. The occupational therapist also assesses sensory, perceptual, motor, and behavioral/emotional impairments (as do physical therapists and speech-language pathologists). Occupational therapists are generally more concerned with how the person takes in information about the world and makes sense of it (sensory input and integration) as well as how the person puts together different perceptions and movements. Self-care skills require fine motor and perceptual abilities and are therefore often addressed by an O.T. Special adaptive equipment the client requires to complete all or part of a self-care task is generally ordered or created by the occupational therapist. Hand or arm braces or splints are also fabricated by the O.T.

Communication disorders are assessed and treated primarily by the *speech-language pathologist.* Evaluation of receptive language (understanding of language) and expressive language (production skills) as well as oral-motor functioning (speech and eating skills related to the structure and function of the oral mechanism) are within this professional's realm. The examination of the oral mechanism includes such structures as the lips, jaw, tongue, palate, teeth, and how well they are used in communication and for eating. Additionally, respiration, voice, and fluency in speech and language are assessed. The speech-language pathologist works with an audiologist to plan treatment for hearing difficulties or to determine whether amplification—such as an auditory trainer or hearing aids—is needed. The speech-language pathologist is often the contact person for communication boards or devices, including switch mechanisms or augmentative/alternative communication aids. (Augmentative/ alternative communication refers to any system a person can use to help with communication.)

For all types of therapy, after an evaluation has been completed, the therapist then recommends a treatment plan. This plan can include individual or small-group treatment, staff-directed programming after inservice training, or other ways of delivering treatment. It is essential that the client's treatment be coordinated across all settings where the individual spends time, not only at home, but at a school or work setting as well.

In summary, current trends in the care of clients with developmental disabilities include the following:

- Clients are being moved out of institutions into small, individualized residential settings.
- Clients participate in active treatment during daily-care activities.
- Clients experience greater participation in the community.
- Treatment goals emphasize clients' abilities/strengths.
- Clients' needs are managed by an interdisciplinary team.

Each person—from the client to the direct-care staff—plays an integral part in the management process. The crucial elements of habilitation are promoting each individual's independence and integration into society.

2
Muscle Tone and Handling Techniques

Daily handling of an individual with multiple disabilities can, at first glance, seem overwhelmingly complex. A basic understanding of the pathology or origin of the disability will help you to become an efficient and beneficial caregiver for clients. This chapter will discuss *cerebral palsy,* which is often the disorder underlying the individual's disabilities. You will learn the different physical characteristics resulting from cerebral palsy that you will observe as you are caring for people. By learning how to provide "handling with understanding," you can positively affect the disabled individual's daily life experiences.

Cerebral palsy is a disorder resulting from damage to the brain occurring at or around the time of birth. It can be caused by bleeding in the brain tissue, by abnormal brain development, or by lack of sufficient oxygen to brain structures. This damage to the brain causes incorrect information to be transmitted or relayed from the brain to the muscles of the body. The result is abnormal *muscle tone,* which in turn causes problems with movement. Muscle tone is the tension or resistance present in our muscles at all times. Normal muscle tone enables us to "hold" our bodies in proper alignment as we move and as we rest.

Severe cases of cerebral palsy are usually apparent within the first months of life. Cerebral palsy is not progressive. A child may appear to worsen with time, however, because as the person exerts greater effort to move, the movements appear more and more abnormal.

Abnormal muscle tone caused by cerebral palsy can be manifested in different ways and in different body parts depending on the area of the brain that is affected. The three basic types of abnormal muscle tone are *hypertonicity, hypotonicity,* and *fluctuating muscle tone.*

Hypertonicity

Hypertonicity or spasticity is described as increased resistance to passive movement. Hypertonicity can be present in muscles that flex (bend) and those that extend (straighten) the arms, legs, and trunk. It can also occur in the muscles that pull the limbs toward the center of the body (adduction and internal rotation).

For example, if a person's elbow is spastic or hypertonic into flexion you will feel resistance when you try to straighten or extend it. If the legs are spastic or hypertonic into adduction and extension, you will feel resistance when you try to bend the knees and open the legs. Spasticity can be present in all parts of the body including the face, neck, back, abdomen, wrist, fingers, ankles, and toes.

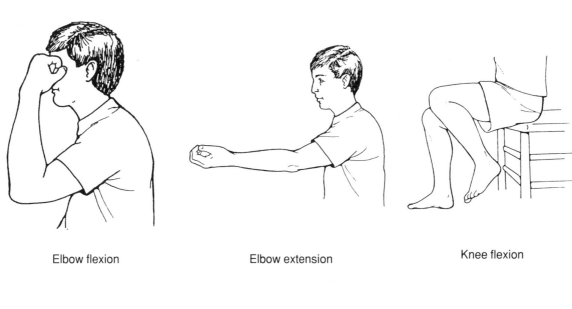

Elbow flexion

Elbow extension

Knee flexion

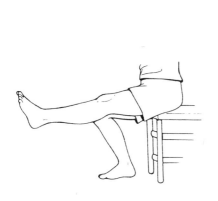

Knee extension

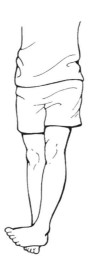

Adduction and internal rotation of the leg

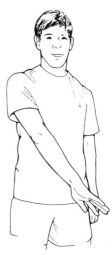

Adduction and internal rotation of the arm

Hypotonicity

Hypotonicity is described as decreased resistance to passive movement. Hypotonic individuals have a "floppy" or "rag doll-like" feel to their arms, legs, and trunk. They tend to collapse where gravity "pulls" them. For example, they often have difficulty holding their heads up or holding their backs straight. Their legs and arms fall easily out and away from the body. The muscles in their faces are frequently involved, creating varying degrees of speech and feeding difficulties.

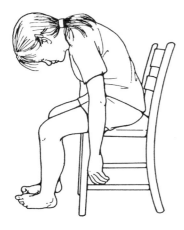

Hypotonia in sitting

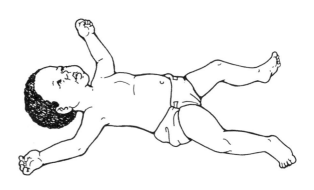

Hypotonia in back lying

Fluctuating Muscle Tone

Fluctuating muscle tone changes from hypotonic to hypertonic and is often accompanied by uncontrolled movement. Persons with fluctuating muscle tone look unbalanced and unsteady when they try to move. For example, as they reach for an object they may stiffen into extension and then quickly collapse into flexion.

Types of Cerebral Palsy

Cerebral palsy is classified according to the parts of the body affected by the specific brain centers that have been damaged. Each type can mildly, moderately, or severely affect the person, depending on the amount of damage the brain has sustained.

Spastic diplegia

Spastic diplegia affects the lower parts of the body more than the upper parts. Persons with this type of cerebral palsy are generally able to use their hands and arms to help themselves to function. They are quite often able to learn to walk alone or with the help of a walker or crutches. Walking, though, continues to require excessive effort. These individuals are usually able to speak and take care of their daily needs.

Spastic hemiplegia

Spastic hemiplegia is a type of cerebral palsy characterized by abnormal movement and control primarily on one side of the body. Usually both the arm and leg on the affected side are hypertonic. Balance reactions in that direction are absent or diminished, causing the hemiplegic individual to rely on the opposite side of the body; these individuals may look as though they are "ignoring" the affected side during motor tasks. Speech is usually present; walking is often very functional and without extreme effort.

Spastic quadriplegia

Spastic quadriplegia cerebral palsy involves the entire body. All the limbs are spastic, and control of the trunk and head is very poor. Many times, one side of the body is more hypertonic than the other. Muscle tone often fluctuates. Severe feeding and speech problems are common. This is the most severe type of cerebral palsy and is probably the type most frequently seen in institutional and group-home settings, where clients are entirely dependent on others for their daily needs.

It should be noted here that, because the brain is responsible for so many aspects of our daily functioning, cerebral palsy often affects more than a person's ability to move. There is frequently overlap and involvement in areas responsible for sensation, perception, vision, hearing, and all types of learning and intellectual processes. Problems in these areas will be discussed in later chapters.

The following sections describe techniques for effectively handling individuals who are hypotonic and hypertonic. The handling techniques you will learn for hypertonicity and hypotonicity can be used in combination for persons with fluctuating muscle tone.

Handling the Hypertonic Client

Individuals who are severely hypertonic or spastic do not have a range of intricate, planned, voluntary movements available to them. Instead they tend to move reflexively (see chapter 4) in mass, stereotyped patterns. It is difficult for them to move one part of the body independently of another part.

Illustrations of this concept include the following:

Bending the hip while straightening the knee

Normally an individual is able to straighten the knee and remain in a sitting position. When a person with extensor spasticity straightens the knee, however, the hip straightens as well. This reduces stability and the ability to maintain a sitting position.

Extensor spasticity results in difficulty maintaining a sitting position.

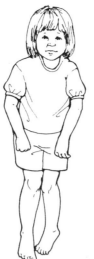

Keeping the foot flat while straightening the hip and knee to stand

In normal standing the foot remains flat, keeping the upright body balanced. As the spastic leg straightens and bears weight, the ankle straightens and the toes point down, making the base of support for the body too small for adequate balance.

Problems in standing may be due to a small base of support.

Raising the head in stomach lying while supported on bent elbows

In the *prone* or stomach lying position, an individual with spasticity has difficulty raising or lifting the head and neck while supporting the weight of the body on flexed elbows. Instead the head stays down, making movement more difficult. Spasticity in the shoulders also keeps the elbows back so they cannot come forward to adequately support weight.

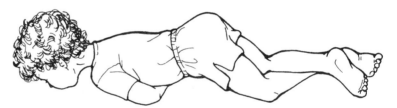

This child is unable to raise the head in stomach lying.

Spastic movement of the legs and arms tends to follow patterns that do not allow for normal postural alignment of the body. These patterns interfere with day-to-day function. These abnormal patterns occur either into flexion or into extension.

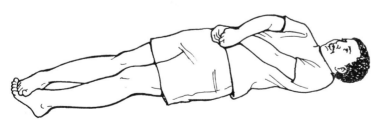

Extensor pattern

Extensor pattern

In the extensor pattern, the arms pull together toward the midline of the body (imagine a line down the center of the body) and the elbows straighten. The legs also pull together (*adduct*), the knees straighten, and the toes point downward.

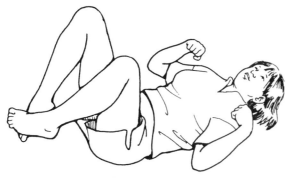

Flexor pattern

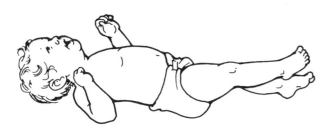

Flexor pattern of the upper body
with extensor pattern of the lower body

Flexor pattern

The flexor pattern pulls the arms and shoulders back. The elbows, wrists, and fingers flex. The hips and knees pull tightly into flexion.

Sometimes a combination of flexion and extension patterns can occur. This is often seen when individuals with spasticity are trying to move. For example, the hands-and-knees position might cause mass extension of the upper body with total flexion of the lower body. In back lying, it is common to see movement combining flexion of the upper body and extension of the lower body, or extension of the upper body with flexion of the lower body.

Tips for Handling a Hypertonic Person

Your approach significantly affects how the hypertonic person responds to the environment. Your good handling will help the person to be able to move more normally. You will notice that stress or overexcitement increases the degree of spasticity. A calm, unhurried approach will keep the person calm. Touch should be firm but gentle, and your own movements should be slow. Light touch and quick movements increase spasticity.

Where you place your hands on the person can greatly inhibit, minimize, or decrease spasticity. Proper hand positioning makes more normal movement possible for your clients and helps them to feel more secure and safe. When you assist a person to move, the most effective points of the body for you to control are closest to the trunk. These include the spine and the pelvic and shoulder girdles. If you are helping someone to roll in bed, for example, put your hand behind the shoulder and bring the upper body toward you. *Never* pull at the lower arm or hand to bring the upper body forward. If you are assisting a person in moving the lower body, support the area around the hip and move the hip forward or back. Don't pull or push at the lower leg.

Your hand should hold the person over as large a surface area as possible. Spread your fingers to provide gentle support with the entire palm of your hand.

Decreasing Spasticity

Spasticity can be inhibited or decreased by holding the spastic body part in patterns opposite to those of the dominating spastic patterns. In the flexor pattern, spasticity pulls the shoulder back and the elbow and wrist into flexion. To counteract the flexor pattern, put your hand behind the shoulder and bring it forward. Then gently and slowly straighten the elbow and bring the arm out and away from the body with the wrist and hand facing up.

In the extensor pattern, the legs are extended at the hip, knee, and ankle. To help break up this spastic pattern, flex the hip and knee. Control of the head is often a problem for individuals with cerebral palsy. The neck can thrust the head back into extension or make the head fall forward into flexion. Be certain when positioning or moving your clients that their heads are well supported and not allowed to fall forward or backward or to the side.

The more normal you can make a movement feel for the person you care for, the better the individual will be able to reproduce that movement independently. Normal movement patterns experienced again and again inhibit spastic, hypertonic muscles and make functional, directed movement more likely.

Rolling movement of the lower part of the body near the hips is called *rotation*. Rotation tends to be relaxing and has the effect of reducing spasticity. The relaxation technique illustrated makes use of rotation and can be incorporated into your daily routine with hypertonic individuals.

Relaxation Technique Using Rotation

1. With the individual in back lying, slowly and gently bend the hips and knees toward the body. Keep the client's head in the center or midline of the body. Your hands should be on the knees, guiding the movement and keeping the knees apart.

2. Then slowly and gently move both legs as a unit to the left, and then to the right. Repeat this until you feel the legs and body relax.

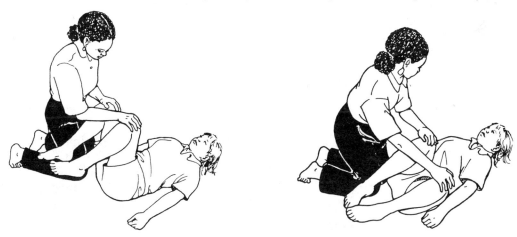

These two illustrations show the rotation technique.

Slowly and *gently* are key words; remember that spastic muscles respond to quick, hard movements by becoming more spastic. Slow, gentle movements inhibit or relax spastic, hypertonic muscles. This simple exercise can precede diaper changing, bathing, dressing, and positioning in equipment. It will help your clients to be more comfortable and relaxed as they are handled. Rotation should also be incorporated in moving individuals from one position to another. When moving a person from back lying to sitting, bend the hips and knees toward the chest. Roll the person into sidelying and bring the legs over the side of the bed. As you give support behind the bottom shoulder and in front of the top hip, help the person assume a sitting position. Never pull on the arms or legs or pull the person straight up from back lying. Support the shoulder girdle and the hips and make use of rotation. Give support to the head if needed. (How to use rotation to aid in dressing and undressing a client is illustrated in chapter 9.)

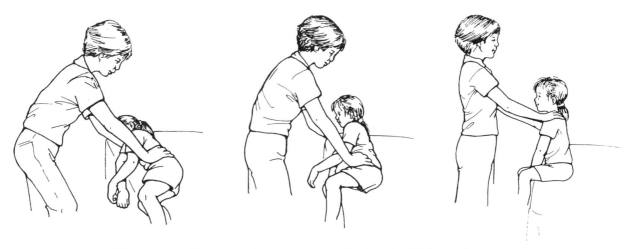

This sequence illustrates using rotation in moving from back lying to sitting.

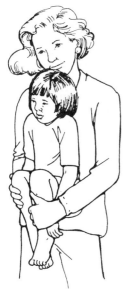

Lifting a child

Transferring and Lifting

With children or adults who are small enough to be carried, the effects of spasticity can be minimized by the manner in which they are carried. Smaller clients can be carried with their backs to you. The legs should be flexed and the knees held apart. Make sure the head does not fall forward or backward or to the side.

Larger clients who need to be totally assisted to move from one place to another can be moved or carried by two people in a similar manner. Support the shoulder girdle and hips. Keep your bodies close to the client's body, taking care to keep the head in good alignment.

It is important that you protect your own body while lifting heavy clients. Improper lifting can tire and injure your back. The muscles in your back are small and are easily strained by heavy loads. Your legs have large, heavy muscle groups that are better designed to do the work required in lifting. Before lifting someone, check to make sure your body is as close as possible to the body of the person and that your back is straight. Next, bend your knees to get into the desired position for lifting. Then lift by straightening your legs. Do not bend over to pick someone up. Many times, it is better to use two people to lift clients. This is especially true when handling larger individuals. A client's safety should never be compromised. If you have any doubt that you will be able to lift a client alone, ask for help from another person. Two-person carries are illustrated in chapter 9.

The act of moving from one position or piece of equipment to another is referred to as a *transfer*. Some clients will need less assistance from you to transfer than others. The amount of assistance given to the individual can be classified as *minimal, moderate,* or *maximum.*

Minimal assistance. Giving minimal assistance means guiding the client's movement with your hand position and providing your strength only during parts of the transfer the client can't independently perform. If a client can transfer independently and understands simple commands, you may be able to stand close by to offer help as needed. Help could include gentle guiding with your hands or verbal cues.

Moderate assistance. With moderate assistance, you provide support to the body parts being moved. You do part of the work, while allowing your client to participate in the movement as much as possible.

Maximum assistance. Maximum assistance means that you provide the strength and movement from your own body to transfer the client from one place to another.

The following illustrations show a wheelchair-to-bed transfer called a *pivot transfer*. It would be used with a person who is capable of helping with the transfer. Position the wheelchair close to and angled toward the bed. This results in the shortest possible distance between the bed and the chair. Lock the brakes of the wheelchair. Stand in front of the person, blocking the feet and knees with your own feet and knees. Bring the upper body forward, bending the hips. Put your hand behind the client's

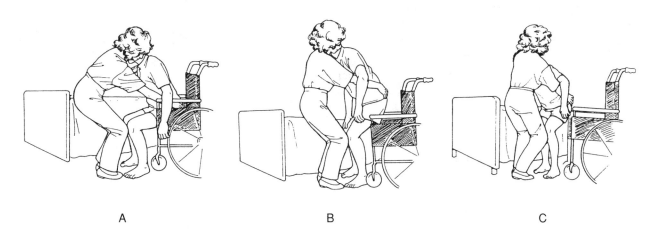

A   B   C

The pivot transfer from a wheelchair to a bed.

shoulder. Put your other hand on the back of the pelvis and help the person to come forward and take weight on the feet. Once standing, help the person to turn by pivoting (turning) and guiding the hips toward the bed. Keep the upper body forward and slowly help the individual to lower to the bed. If the person is lying in bed and needs to transfer to a wheelchair, use the rotation technique described previously to bring the client to sitting. Place the feet flat on the floor, directly under the knees, and slightly apart. Then complete the pivot transfer as just described.

More independent individuals often need assistance to move from a standing position to the floor. Have the person stabilize by holding onto the arms of a chair or a low piece of furniture with both hands. Be sure to use a heavy piece that won't tip or slide under the person's weight. Shift the person's weight onto one leg. Help to bend the nonsupporting knee, keeping the hip straight and the knee directly under the hip. Then help to lower the nonsupporting knee to the floor slowly. This position is called *half-kneeling*. From half-kneeling, bring the other knee to the floor. Then help the client to assume the hands-and-knees position. The hips can then be brought down and to the side into a side-sitting position. This transfer assumes that the client is capable of independent, directed movement.

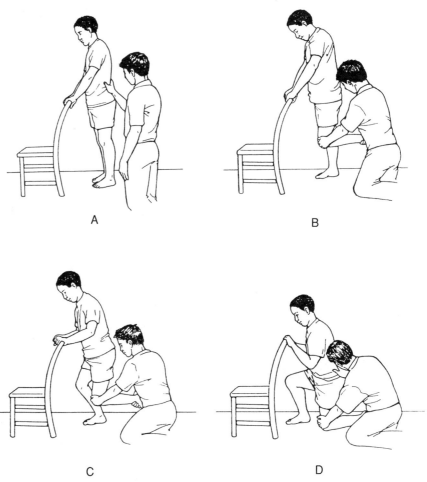

This sequence illustrates assisting a client from standing to the floor.

Handling the Hypotonic Client

Hypotonic or floppy individuals need support from you for parts of their bodies over which they have little voluntary control. Remember that gravity works on floppy body parts by pulling them toward the earth. The spine rounds and the legs and arms fall away from the body. The large muscles around joints—which are responsible for holding the body and its parts against gravity—are not functioning properly due to incorrect signals from the damaged brain.

Handling hypotonic individuals seems, at first glance, to be less complicated than caring for persons with hypertonicity. It is difficult, though, to give enough support from your own body without giving so much that the clients don't use the movement and control of which they are capable. The transfer techniques illustrated for hypertonic individuals are applicable to the hypotonic person as well.

Approximation

An additional technique you can use with hypotonia is called *approximation*. Whereas rotation inhibits or relaxes hypertonicity, approximation helps to facilitate or encourage better muscle control from a floppy person. Approximation is pressure applied through joint surfaces. Joints are the areas where segments of the body come together. The pressure should be firm but gentle and should be repeated several times. This is a good technique to use before positioning clients in equipment or before feeding or dressing. It will help to encourage more active movement from your client.

Approximation for the legs

With the person in back lying, support the top of one knee with one hand and cup the heel in your other hand. The hip, knee, and ankle should be at right angles to each other. Push gently down on the knee. This will put pressure through the hip joint. At the same time, push up gently through the heel, putting pressure through the knee and ankle joint. Repeat on the opposite side.

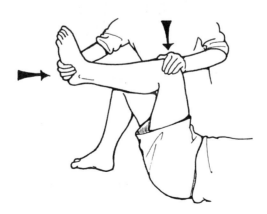

Approximation for the legs

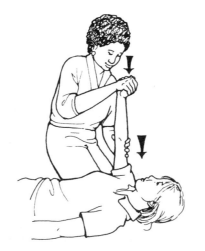

Approximation for the arms

To approximate the arms, position the person in back lying. Hold the person's hand in your own with the wrist extended. Support the elbow with your other hand to keep it straight. Gently apply pressure downward through the entire length of the arm.

Approximation for the arms

Approximation for other body parts

Gently bouncing in sitting will approximate the joints of the back and will facilitate straighter sitting. When holding hypotonic individuals, try to use your body to help them hold the back straight and the head up. Keep their arms and legs from falling away from the body. Use gentle approximation through the back, arms, and legs while you are holding them. The same principles can be applied to larger persons as they are positioned in equipment or as you are helping them move from one place to another.

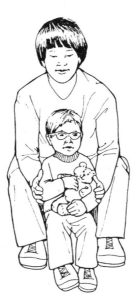

Support a child like this

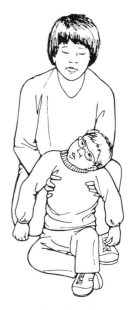

Not like this

If you provide individuals who are disabled with good handling day after day, it will help them to achieve the most normal movement patterns they are capable of. They will also be more comfortable and able to more actively participate in and interact with their environment.

3
Range of Motion

Range of motion describes the arcs of movement that are possible in all the joints of the body. People with normal muscle tone are able to voluntarily move their arms, legs, backs, and necks in the full range of motion possible for each particular joint. Individuals with cerebral palsy have difficulty moving their bodies and limbs voluntarily. Their caretakers need to exercise their bodies for them, so that they can experience full range of motion. If range of motion is not regularly provided for them, muscular shortening and tightening can develop over time, leading to permanent deformities of the bone. If this occurs, movement of the joint is no longer possible.

Range of Motion for the Hypotonic Client

Hypotonic individuals generally have excessive range of motion. Their joints need to be protected because the muscles around them are slack and don't provide normal stabilizing forces to properly hold the joints together. Hypotonic individuals often develop excessive rounding of the back because they are unable to hold their spines straight. It is important for you to provide them with experiences of holding their spines straight in back lying, stomach lying, and sitting. Attention to normal arm and leg position is also very important (see chapter 6).

Never pull hypotonic individuals by the arms or legs to sit them up or to move them. Joints that have poor muscular stabilization can be injured by pulling forces. The neck and the head need good support, especially if the head tends to fall forward or back.

Remember the importance of careful range of motion as it relates to your clients' future state of well-being. You will be contributing to their comfort and may be saving them painful surgical corrections later.

Range of Motion for the Hypertonic Client

Recall from chapter 2 how individuals with hypertonicity move in abnormal patterns of flexion and extension. The muscles that move the body over and over in these same patterns become tight and restrict movement in the opposite direction. Movement can also become restricted because these individuals spend much of their day seated in wheelchairs. Muscle groups that are particularly susceptible to tightening are the following:

- Those that bend the knees
- Those that bend the hips
- Those that pull the toes and ankles down
- Those that pull the legs together and in
- Those that bend the elbows
- Those that bend the wrist
- Those that close the fingers and pull the thumbs in
- Those that pull the shoulders up and back

Range of motion exercises should be performed daily to counteract the effects of hypertonicity (spasticity). Remember that hypertonicity shortens muscles with time. Your efforts will help your clients to fight the battle against time. Range of motion exercises done correctly can help prevent excessive muscle shortening, bony deformities, and even dislocation of joints. These problems may occur even with good daily range of motion, but without it they surely will. If a person has had a surgical procedure to lengthen a tight muscle or to correct a bony deformity, range of motion exercises will be very important to keep the length gained by the surgery. The physician and the consulting therapist will decide when the time is right for you to resume range of motion exercises after surgery.

Many people will be able to assist with their own range of motion exercises. You should encourage them to do so, both verbally and by guiding them through the correct movement patterns. Exercise is always more beneficial if at least part of it can be performed independently. Range of motion can be classified as *active, active assistive,* and *passive.*

Active range of motion. Active range of motion means that the client can do the majority of the movement independently. All that is needed from you is guidance by verbal instruction and by helping the client to move the body part in the desired pattern.

Active assistive range of motion. Active assistive range of motion requires that you provide the movement for the individual during the parts of the pattern that cannot be done independently. In other words, you add your strength to the client's, allowing the person as much voluntary control as possible.

Passive range of motion. Passive range of motion means that, due to abnormal muscle tone or abnormal reflexive responses, the client cannot contribute independent movement to the exercise pattern. The movement of the body part is provided entirely by you.

Range of motion should be done slowly. Give the part of the body you are moving good support with your own body. A good rule to remember is to give support above the joint you are moving. For example, support the upper arm while you move the elbow. Support the lower leg while you move the ankle. Move the limb to the point where you feel resistance, and then gently hold the body part at that point. Range of motion should *not* be painful. If it hurts, you have gone too far. You will often feel a spastic (hypertonic) muscle relaxing more as you hold it, making it possible then to move the joint a small distance farther. When you release the body part, let go *slowly.* A spastic muscle acts much like a rubber band. If you release it too quickly, it will "spring back" to its shortened position. Repeat range of motion exercises several times for maximum benefit.

Before beginning range of motion with a particular client, consult with the physical therapist or occupational therapist who visits your setting so that a specialist can review and demonstrate the following illustrated exercises for you. The therapist will also tell you which patterns of movement to use with individual clients. Use this manual for a guideline only after you have been personally instructed.

The following pages are reproducible for inclusion in the client's daily-care plan.

Range of Motion for the Legs

The Hip

The hip joint is capable of six movements: flexion, extension, abduction, adduction, internal rotation, and external rotation. In spasticity, the muscles that bend (flex) the hip and the muscles that pull the leg in toward the midline of the body (adduct) are often tight. The following hip exercises work best with the individual in back lying. Placing the person in the stomach lying position, though, is useful for passively stretching the hip joint into extension, especially for individuals who spend much of their day in a wheelchair.

To flex the hip, put one hand on the front of the knee with the other hand cupping the heel. The ankle should be at a right angle to the lower leg. Don't allow the knee to pull in (adduct). Bend the hip so the knee comes up toward the chest. To extend the hip, reverse the movement, straightening the hip and knee.

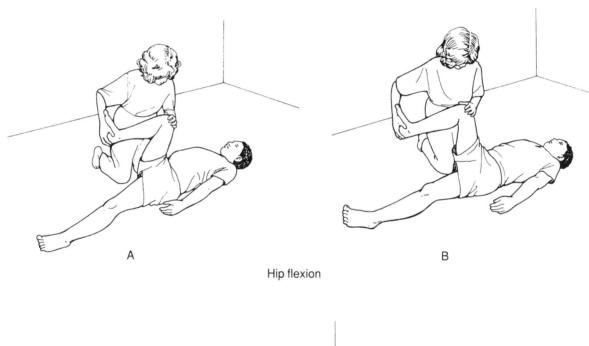

A   B

Hip flexion

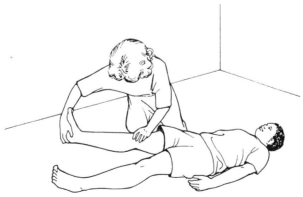

Hip extension

To abduct the hip, move the leg away from the midline of the body by placing one hand on the top and inside of the knee and the other hand on the top and outside of the hip. The muscles on the inside of the leg are often tight. Hold the leg in this position to stretch these muscles. Adduct—that is, move the leg back—just to the midpoint of the body.

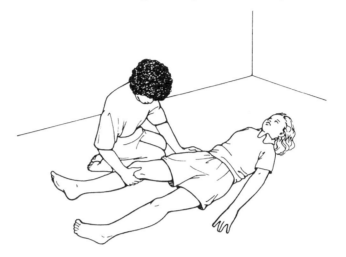

Hip abduction

To externally rotate the hip joint, place one hand on the top and inside of the knee and the other hand on the top and outside of the hip. The knee should be slightly flexed. Rotate the upper leg by moving the knee so it faces away from the body. Internally rotate the hip back to the starting position until the knee points straight up.

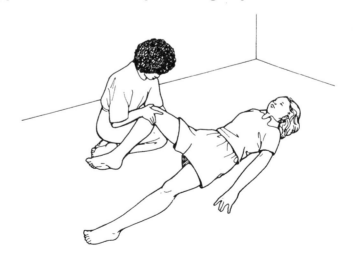

Hip external rotation

The Knee

The knee is capable of just two movements: flexion and extension. Range of motion for the knee can be done in back lying, sitting, or stomach lying. Knee extension (straightening) is difficult for the individual with spasticity, especially in the sitting position, as the muscle behind the knee is often tight.

To extend the knee, place one hand on the top of the knee. Cup the heel in your other hand. Straighten the knee. Hold this straightened position to stretch the muscles behind the knee. Then bend (flex) the knee in the opposite direction.

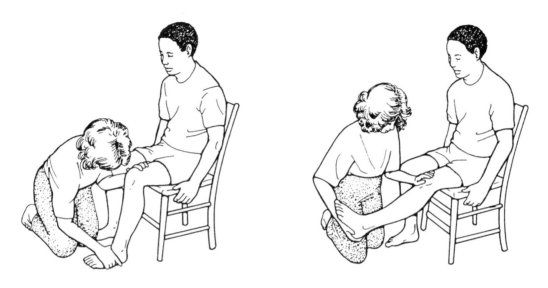

Knee flexion and extension in sitting

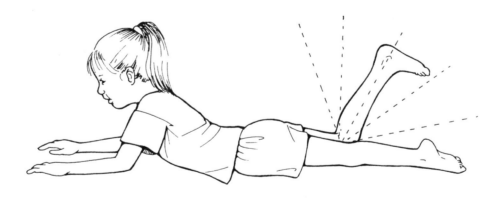

Knee flexion and extension may work better in stomach lying
with people who have a greater degree of spasticity.

Copyright © 1991 by Cindy French, Robin Tapp González, and Jan Tronson-Simpson
Published by Therapy Skill Builders, a division of The Psychological Corporation. All rights reserved.
1-800-211-8378 / ISBN 0761647058

The Ankle

The feet and ankles are easiest to move in the sitting position with the client well supported. The ankle joint is capable of moving up and down and in and out. Individuals with spasticity tend to have tightness in the muscles behind the lower leg, which keeps their feet pointed downward. It is very important to keep these muscles from tightening; if the muscles permanently shorten, it is impossible to bear weight on the feet properly.

To move the ankle up, place one hand in a cupped position behind the heel. Put your other hand under the foot, supporting the arch on the inside of the foot. Avoid putting pressure on the ball of the foot. Too much pressure here can stimulate abnormal reflexes and cause damage to the tissues of the feet. Push up on the bottom of the foot; at the same time pull down on the back of the heel. Take care to keep the foot in good alignment.

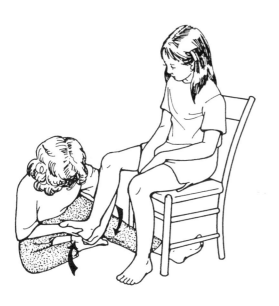

Moving the ankle

The Toes

The toes can be straightened (extended) and bent (flexed). With spasticity, the toes often "claw" into flexion. This can be diminished or inhibited by gently straightening and pulling the toes up. Abnormal muscle tone can also pull the toes toward the inside or outside of the foot, which can cause pain and joint deformity. Hold the foot and ankle in a properly aligned position. Align the toes as much as possible. With the other hand under the toes, gently move them up and down.

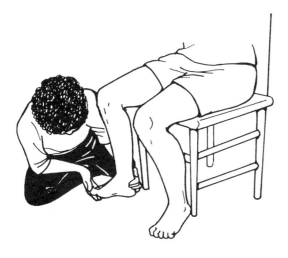

Extension of the toes

Range of Motion for the Arms

The arms are most easily exercised in back lying, unless the person is able to sit alone. In back lying, the surface the client is lying on provides support to the back and shoulder girdle. With this support the individual is more likely to be able to perform part of the range of motion pattern independently. If a client is able to sit without support and has good control of the head the exercises can be done in a sitting position in a sturdy chair with the feet well stabilized on the floor or a footrest.

The Shoulder

The shoulder joint is capable of six movements: flexion, extension, abduction, adduction, external rotation, and internal rotation. The entire shoulder girdle can also move up and down (elevating and depressing) and forward and back. The client with spasticity often has tightness in the muscles that pull the shoulders in toward the center of the body (adduct) and in the muscles that elevate and pull the shoulders back. The shoulder is very complicated mechanically and needs to be handled carefully.

To flex the shoulder, put one hand behind the shoulder and the other hand behind the elbow. Hold the elbow straight and the palm of the hand facing up. Keeping the shoulder well supported with your hand, move the arm straight up over the head. The shoulder extends as the arm comes down to the supporting surface. The joint can be further extended by rolling the client onto the side.

Shoulder flexion

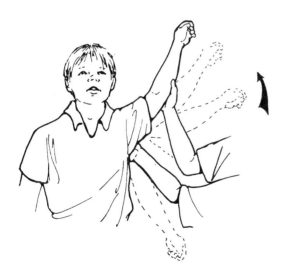

Shoulder abduction

To abduct the shoulder, the arm is brought away from the midpoint of the body. Support with one hand behind the client's shoulder and the other hand behind and to the inside of the elbow. With the palm of the hand facing up and the elbow straight, move the arm in an arc out and away from the body until the arm is above the head. Hold the arm in this position to stretch the muscle that pulls the arm in. Adduct the arm by bringing it back toward the body until the arm rests at the side.

To rotate the shoulder joint, place the client's arm straight out at a right angle to the side of the body. Bend the elbow. Cup your hand behind and to the inside of the elbow, and hold the client's hand with the wrist supported in yours. Bring the hand toward the supporting surface. This is external rotation, often a difficult motion for the client with spasticity. Hold this position to stretch the tight muscles. Then bring the palm of the hand down to the supporting surface. This is internal rotation.

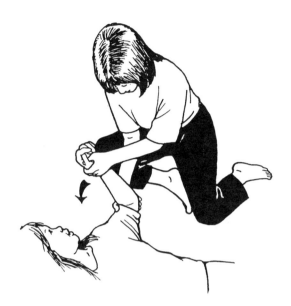

Shoulder external rotation

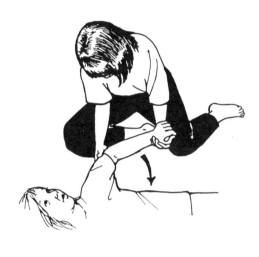

Shoulder internal rotation

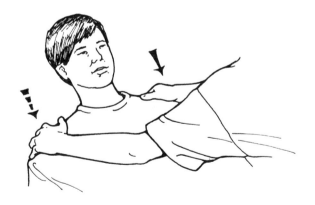

Relaxing the shoulders

Spasticity tends to pull the shoulders up toward the head (elevation) and back toward the spine. Before and after range of motion for the shoulder joint, it is helpful to work with the shoulder girdle to bring the shoulders down and forward. Put your hands on the top of both shoulders with your fingers cupped behind the shoulder blades. One at a time, bring the shoulders gently down and forward, repeating this alternating movement until you feel the shoulders relax.

Published by Therapy Skill Builders, a division of The Psychological Corporation. All rights reserved.
1-800-211-8378 / ISBN 0761647058

The Elbow

The elbow joint is capable of two motions: flexion and extension. Tightness commonly develops in the muscles that flex (bend) the elbow. The muscles of the lower arm also move the arm so that the hand faces upward (palm up) or downward (palm down). Spasticity is common in the muscles that turn the palm downward.

To straighten (extend) the elbow, cup one hand behind the elbow. Place the other hand in front of the wrist. Slowly straighten the arm, holding it in this position to stretch the muscles that bend the elbow. Then bend the elbow, bringing the hand toward the shoulder.

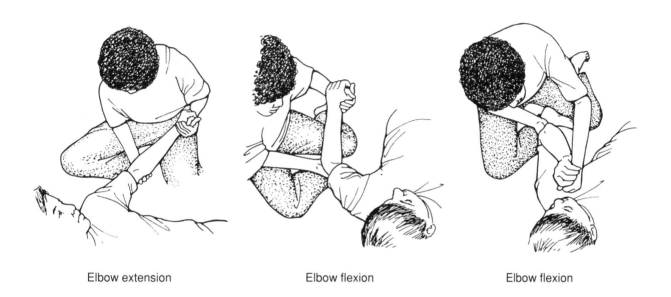

| Elbow extension | Elbow flexion | Elbow flexion |

With one hand behind the elbow and the other holding the person's hand and supporting the wrist, turn the lower arm so the hand is facing up.

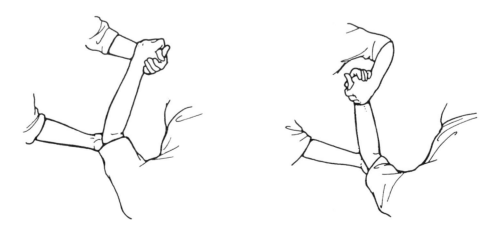

Moving the lower arm to a palm-up position

The Wrist

The wrist joint is capable of flexion (bending), extension (straightening), and of side-to-side movement (toward the little-finger side of the hand and toward the thumb side of the hand). It is common for spasticity to hold the wrist in flexion.

To extend the wrist, support the lower arm below the back of the elbow. Hold the client's hand with your hand and bring the hand up. To flex the wrist, bring the hand down. Then align the wrist with the lower arm, and move the wrist toward the little-finger side of the hand. Then move the wrist toward the thumb side of the hand.

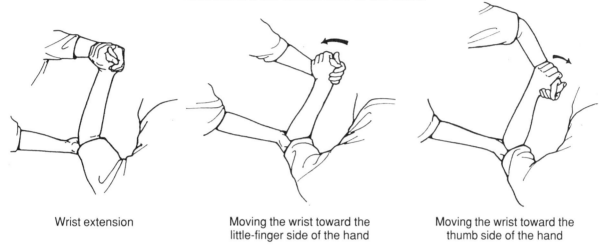

Wrist extension

Moving the wrist toward the little-finger side of the hand

Moving the wrist toward the thumb side of the hand

The Fingers and Thumb

Spasticity tends to pull the fingers into flexion and the thumb in toward the palm of the hand. An effective way of straightening the fingers and bringing the thumb away from the palm is to hold the client's hand in a handshake position. In this manner, the fingers and thumb can be put into a normal position without causing damage to the delicate structures of the hand. *Never* pull at the ends of the fingers or thumb to straighten them. Turning the palm up and putting the wrist into some extension will also aid finger and thumb opening.

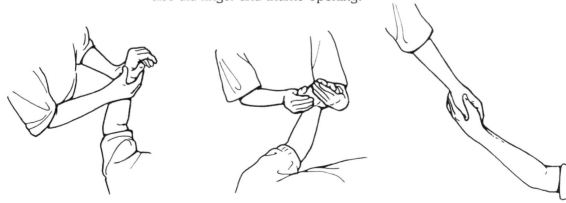

Finger and thumb opening

The handshake position

Considerations for the Neck and Spine

The neck and spine contain many small joints that allow forward, backward, side-to-side, and rotary movements. Due to abnormal muscle tone and abnormal reflexive responses (see chapter 4) the spine is at risk for developing muscular shortening and bony deformity. *Scoliosis* (abnormal side bending of the spine) and *kyphosis* (abnormal forward bending of the spine) are common problems in individuals with abnormal muscle tone. During range of motion exercises, the head should be in line with the back, and the back should be straight. Spasticity often thrusts the head back, tightening the muscles at the back of the neck. Bring the head slightly forward during exercise time by placing a small pillow or towel roll behind the client's head to keep it forward.

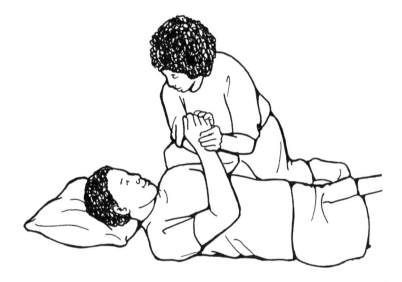

4

Influence of Abnormal Reflexes

In chapter 2 the way movements of hypertonic individuals occur in mass patterns was discussed. These stereotyped patterns limit planned, voluntary movement and are accompanied by abnormal muscle tone. Remember that cerebral palsy results from damage to the brain and that the brain controls planned movement. When damaged, the brain is unable to do its job of providing the muscles with information to make normal movement possible. Instead, abnormal, reflexive, involuntary, unplanned movement occurs. Three reflexes often become abnormally strong after damage to the brain. They occur as the neck and head are moved. It is important for you to have a basic understanding of these abnormal reflexive responses because with proper handling and positioning, their effects can be diminished. Although reflexive responses are not usually strong in hypotonic individuals, proper positioning and handling are important considerations for them as well (see chapters 2 and 6).

Reflexive Responses

ATNR

ATNR stands for *asymmetrical tonic neck reflex.* Asymmetry means that one side of the body looks different from the other. As the head turns to one side, the arm and leg on the opposite side bend, and the arm and leg on the face side of the head straighten. This response can occur as the head is turned to the right or to the left.

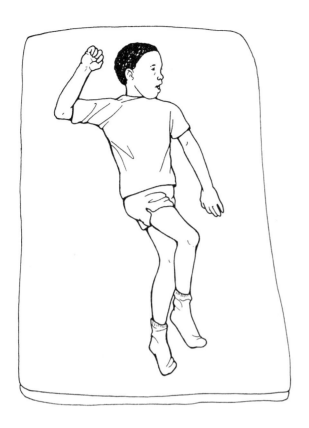

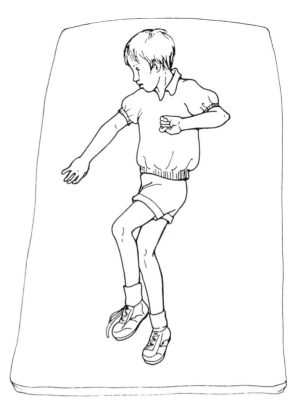

ATNR to the left   ATNR to the right

The ATNR interferes with bringing the hands together and with bringing the arm and leg across the body for rolling. When you are working with a client, try to keep the head at the midline of the body whenever possible. The midline head position decreases the influence of the ATNR and will make it easier for you to feed, dress, exercise, and move your clients. It will also help them to more actively participate in activities of daily care.

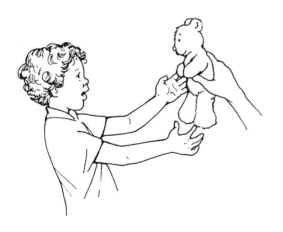

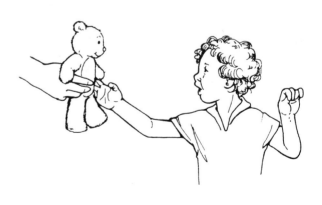

Hand objects to clients in midline   Not to one side

STNR

STNR stands for *symmetrical tonic neck reflex.* Symmetrical means "the same." The STNR is usually associated with attempted movement from one place to another. As the neck bends bringing the head forward, both arms bend and both legs straighten. As the neck straightens and brings the head back, both arms straighten and both legs bend.

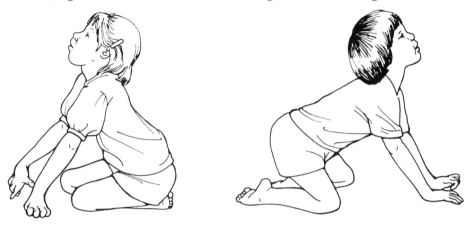

STNR in sitting   STNR on hands and knees

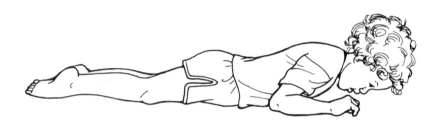

STNR in stomach lying

The STNR interferes with reciprocal (back and forth) movement of the arms and legs, as occurs in creeping and walking. It also interferes with straightening the neck while bending the arms (a movement you use when bearing weight on the elbows and lifting the head up in stomach lying). It also interferes with bending the neck while straightening the arms (for example, when looking at and reaching for food on a wheelchair tray).

Many individuals with hypertonicity learn to move using the STNR. For example, children with the STNR may move on hands and knees using a "bunny hopping" pattern, rather than creeping forward with one leg and arm at a time. They extend the neck, which extends and straightens both arms. Then both legs are pulled forward together in flexion, moving the individual forward. Clients who have a strong STNR have difficulty moving one leg or arm at a time and need help to learn to move reciprocally. Work with them on hands and knees to bring one arm and leg forward at a time. If this is too difficult, turn them on their backs and help them to bring one knee to the chest while keeping the other leg straight. Then reverse the movement on the opposite leg.

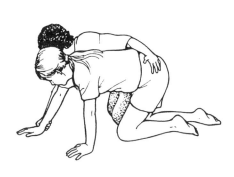

Reciprocal movement of the arms and legs
on hands and knees

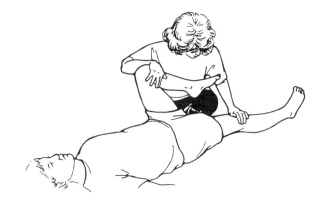

Reciprocal movement of the legs in back lying

In stomach lying, help clients to combine neck straightening with elbow bending, as illustrated below.

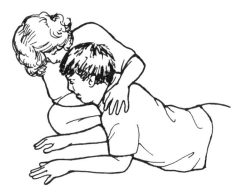

Raising the head while supported on bent elbows inhibits the STNR

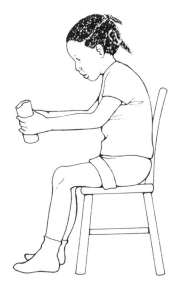

Looking down while reaching
inhibits the STNR

When reaching from a sitting position, help clients to bend the neck while straightening the arm. (Place the object you are handing them in the correct position to encourage this movement.) This will directly oppose the pattern of the STNR.

Tonic Reflex in Back Lying and Stomach Lying

Tonic refers to being "fixed" or stuck in a position. Whereas the STNR depends on neck position during attempted movements, the tonic reflex depends on whether the person is lying face up or face down. More severely involved individuals tend to have strong tonic reflexes. In back lying, the tonic reflex causes the arms and legs to straighten and pull in toward the midline of the body, while the head and shoulders pull back.

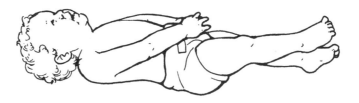

Tonic reflex in back lying

In stomach lying the tonic reflex causes the arms, legs, and head to bend, pulling the body into a ball.

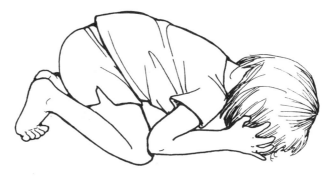

Tonic reflex in stomach lying

The tonic reflex interferes greatly with all movement and functional abilities. Good positioning helps to decrease the influence of this reflex.

In back lying, position the client with the head forward. Flex the hips and knees and bring the shoulders gently forward. Help the hands to come together at midline.

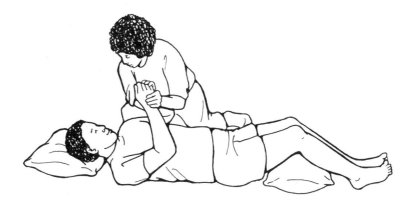

Good positioning in back lying

In stomach lying use a wedge to help the client support weight on the elbows (see chapter 6). In sidelying, place a pillow between the legs to keep them apart and keep the hands at midline.

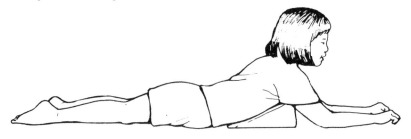

Using a wedge to achieve good positioning in stomach lying

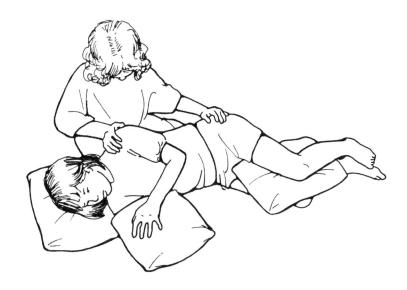

Good positioning in sidelying

In summary, by positioning a person carefully, you can avoid triggering abnormal reflexes. This frees the person for voluntary, purposeful movement. The ATNR causes the arms and legs to flex or extend as the neck is turned from side to side. The STNR causes the arms and legs to flex or extend as the neck is moved forward and backward. The tonic reflex causes the entire body to extend in back lying and to flex in stomach lying. By gently moving the body in directions that oppose these reflexes, you can help diminish their effects.

5
Sensory Impairments

The people you care for will have multiple, interacting handicapping conditions. Frequently, where one abnormality exists, the individual is at increased risk for others. Many of these conditions are visible—the inability to stand or walk, deformities of the hands or feet, or a very large or very small head size. An individual with multiple disabilities may, however, have additional impairments in the senses of vision, hearing, or touch. These deficits may range from mild to severe, and the person may have any combination of these problems. This chapter will give you some general guidelines so you can work more effectively with people who have these conditions. Consulting therapists and outside resource people may also be able to help you with a particular situation.

Visual Impairment

A person may have any degree of visual impairment from a mild loss of vision or *visual field* (the area you can see at one time without turning your head) to total blindness. The damage can be located in the *eye*, in the nerve connections between the eye and the brain, or in the brain itself. Really knowing what or how much people with severe disabilities are able to see is often difficult because they may have difficulty telling us. We must become good observers and try to help our clients "see" in the environment and situations that are best for them. Listed here are some behaviors that might clue you in to how much a person sees. If you suspect an individual thought to be blind has some vision, share your observations with the appropriate resource person. The information may be invaluable.

1. Does the person turn toward or stare at a light source (such as a window)?

2. Does the person appear unusually sensitive to light?

3. Does the person's head frequently tilt a certain way? (This may indicate that the person is compensating for a visual field cut.)

4. Do the person's eyes follow moving objects or people?

5. Does the person squint or close the eyes when the amount of light increases—for example, when going outside after being indoors or when a bright lamp is turned on?

6. Does the person bring objects close to one eye or one side? Does the person look directly at a desired object when reaching rather than out of the corner of one eye?

These are some guidelines for helping individuals who have poor sight:

1. Use other senses to help compensate for the visual loss.

   • When appropriate, encourage clients to touch the objects or people with which they are interacting. If necessary, guide their hands.

   • Describe to clients things sighted people take for granted and talk about how things relate to each other. For example, explain that water can come out of a faucet or spigot, come down as rain or snow, and freeze into ice. Then help them experience the things you talked about.

   • When possible, have the individual move and feel a motion while you describe it. A good example is clapping hands. Young children with visual impairments probably will not know what made the clapping sound—or that they can do it by themselves—unless they have experienced this before.

2. Help the person to realize the parts that go together to create whole objects. Assist the person to touch parts of an object in sequence, while you discuss how the parts are related.

3. Involve the child with limited vision in movement-based activities, just as you would any other child. Remember to maintain good positioning if the child has physical involvement. Always tell the person what you are going to do in advance—especially with activities such as tickling or rocking that can be startling. Then go ahead and have fun.

4. When you choose an activity, try to imagine how much fun it would be without vision. Think about these questions:

- What kind of sound(s) does it produce?

- How does it feel?

- Can the person control or participate in the activity?

5. With individuals who have limited vision or have unknown visual capabilities, here are some things you can do:

- Present items so they contrast with the background. For example, to encourage independent finger feeding, place crackers on a piece of paper or a place mat so the cracker shows up clearly.

- Use good lighting, so the light shines directly on the object.

- Be consistent about the placement of objects and the arrangement of the person's living area. For individuals who can feed themselves, develop a consistent arrangement for utensils and food to encourage independence.

Hearing Impairment

One handicapping condition that is not visible is hearing impairment. Hearing impairment results in a communication disorder that greatly affects quality of life. A person with hearing loss may be deprived of environmental sound experiences and be hindered in developing social relationships.

There are two main types of hearing impairment, and an individual may have one or both types. The first is called an *organic* hearing disorder, meaning that somewhere in the hearing mechanism an identifiable physiological or structural dysfunction causes or contributes to the hearing loss. The second is called a *functional* hearing disorder, meaning that there is no apparent physical cause. Rather, the hearing disorder results from abnormal functioning of the brain. Functional hearing loss implies that the structures of the hearing organ are all working satisfactorily, but the person may have difficulty attaching meaning to sounds. Such people may have good hearing, in that their attention can be aroused by a variety of sounds, but these sounds or words have little or no meaning for them. Suspect a functional hearing loss if your client has difficulty with attention, motivation, and understanding of language.

Maintaining Good Hearing

The following are preventive measures to help maintain good hearing, whether or not the person already has a hearing loss:

1. Follow good *aural* (ear) hygiene rules.

    *   Wash the outside part of the ear routinely during bathing and hair washing.

    *   *Never* stick anything smaller than your elbow in anyone's ear! There is no reason to poke anything into the ear canal, and it's easy to damage the ear drum and bones of the middle ear this way. Ear wax normally works out of the ear by itself. Sometimes, however, the ear canal may become blocked with wax. In this case, it should be removed by a physician.

    *   Contact a medical professional whenever you see any type of discharge or drainage from the ear. This is a sign of ear infection.

2. Each individual should have a yearly hearing test, administered by a trained professional such as an *audiologist,* in order to monitor hearing ability. A hearing test may be part of the individual's annual physical examination.

3. Ear infections may cause significant temporary hearing losses, and repeated ear infections can permanently damage the structures of the ear. It's very important, therefore, that ear infections receive prompt medical attention. Because many of your clients are nonverbal and can't tell you they are in pain, be on the watch for signs of an ear infection. The person may pull at or hit the ears or suddenly become less responsive to sounds, or you may notice discharge from the ear. People with persistent colds or allergies have greater risk of ear infection.

4. Protect the individual's hearing from excessive noise. Sounds that are loud, long-lasting, or repetitive, such as a radio or television turned to high volume, can cause a *noise-induced* hearing loss. (Loud rock music can damage your hearing, as well as your clients'!) A noise-induced loss develops slowly. Once you are aware of it, it is too late to stop it. Be careful when using earphones with a client. Frequently monitor the volume to make sure it hasn't accidentally been turned up.

Communicating with a Person Who Has Hearing Loss

Here are strategies to help a person with a hearing loss better understand you:

1. Try to limit other distractions. It is more difficult to tune in to and understand speech when there is background noise present.

2. Find out whether the person hears better with one ear than the other. If so, speak on the side of the better ear. Also ask the audiologist whether the person has better hearing for high-pitched or low-pitched sounds. It may be helpful to speak in a high voice or a deep, low voice.

3. Always get hearing-impaired people's attention before speaking to them or expecting them to attend to sounds. For instance, you might gently touch or tap the wheelchair or the individual as an attention signal without, you hope, startling the person.

4. Position yourself at close range where you can make eye contact while talking.

5. Speak slowly, clearly, and simply. Remember, even without understanding all your words, individuals will get information through your tone of voice, gestures, and expressions.

6. Use the other senses—vision, touch, and smell—to help the individual make associations with sounds.

7. Every individual should be spoken to or addressed in a respectful manner, regardless of whether the person responds.

Tactile Impairments

Children or adults with any degree of handicapping condition may show either heightened or reduced responses to touch. These two tactile system problems—tactile defensiveness and hyposensitivity—will be described and some general suggestions given.

A person with *tactile defensiveness* has a heightened response to touch. Even though the pressure of your touch feels "normal" to you, the person may feel discomfort and withdraw, become aggressive or more active, or show abnormal movements caused by neurological damage (for example, a person with high muscle tone may fist the hands). For some individuals, routine life experiences may feel uncomfortable or threatening. For example, these individuals might be able to receive hugs they initiate, but find the physical contact too overwhelming when the hug is initiated by someone else. Light touch—for example when lightly patting or guiding someone—may be especially unpleasant. Clients may prefer clothing made of certain types of fabric or may want to wear long sleeves (to reduce the tactile input to their arms) even on a hot day. The individual who refuses to walk barefoot on grass, refuses to eat, or spits out foods of certain textures may be responding to heightened sensations of touch.

Generally, the person will respond better to firm, deep pressure than to light touch. When assisting an individual to walk, for example, guide the person with a firm, direct hold on the hips or shoulders, not a light pat on the back or a gentle pull on one hand. If you suspect that a client has a tactile dysfunction, discuss with the interdisciplinary team the problems you are seeing. The team can give you specific recommendations for individual clients.

Some individuals, on the other hand, show little or no response to touch (*hyposensitivity*). They may respond only to extreme tactile input, such as biting or hitting themselves. They may show little evidence of pain and may laugh when you would expect them to be in pain. They may crave rough play and handling and may need prolonged contact before the input registers with their tactile systems. These individuals may need a varied program to help them receive tactile input, starting, again, with activities that involve deep pressure. Please ask the person's therapist for specific recommendations.

Note that some individuals with hyposensitivity may not be aware of dangerous or harmful situations and may need to be carefully monitored to prevent injury. Examples include eye poking by a blind person (to cause a visual sensation); poking, hitting, or placing objects in the ears (to cause varied auditory sensations); or continual spinning, which can result in seizures.

Sensory system dysfunctions may not be as obvious as physical disorders, yet they can have severe consequences. The senses of vision, hearing, and touch can all be affected, which limits a person's ability to take in information about the world and to interact with other people. By being aware of sensory deficits, you can assist the person in using other senses to compensate, and you may save the person who is hypersensitive to light or touch from added discomfort.

6
Positioning

Individuals with severe disabilities rely on their caretakers to provide them with opportunities to move and change positions. *Adaptive equipment* (wheelchairs, standing frames, sidelyers, and the like) can be very useful in controlling abnormal movement responses and can make possible a wider variety of daily experiences for a person with limited voluntary movement. This chapter will cover individual pieces of equipment and give specific guidelines for their use. You will also learn about problems you may encounter, solutions to these problems, and practical uses and applications for each piece of equipment. Whenever a piece of equipment is not working or does not fit the user well, contact the vendor from whom it was purchased and notify the consulting occupational or physical therapist.

Abnormal muscle tone can lead to deformities of the bones and muscles. Spastic muscles that continuously pull body parts in the same abnormal patterns of movement can actually change the structure of the bones and muscles permanently, requiring surgical correction. Examples might include dislocated hips, curvature of the spine, tightening of the ankle tendons, or excessive rounding of the back and shoulders. Equipment that aligns the client's body more correctly can aid in preventing or decreasing the severity of such deformities.

The abnormal reflexive responses discussed in chapter 4 also contribute to structural problems of the skeletal and muscular systems. The ATNR causes an asymmetrical posture that can result in curvature of the spine. The STNR makes independent movement of the arms and legs difficult and tends to pull the upper back into forward bending. The tonic reflexes pull the entire body into mass flexion or extension patterns, often causing dislocation of the hips and shortening of the muscles and tendons of the spastic muscle groups. Correct positioning in the appropriate equipment decreases the influence of these abnormal reflexes.

Two important general principles when positioning *any* client are *symmetry* and normal *postural alignment* of the body.

Symmetry. Symmetry means that both sides of the body look the same and that the face is centered at the middle of the body (midline). Because abnormal reflexes pull the body into poorly aligned or asymmetrical postures, equipment is needed to help maintain symmetry.

Alignment. Alignment refers to arranging or positioning the body in a straight line. For example, the back should be straight, not curved to the side, front, or back; the feet should be directly under the knees; the toes should be pointing straight ahead.

Although a person with abnormal muscle tone often cannot achieve perfect symmetry and alignment, you should make every attempt to achieve the best possible symmetry and alignment. These guidelines can be applied to persons with increased or decreased muscle tone. Try thinking about how your own body looks when you are sitting, standing, or lying on your stomach. Then try to reproduce these normal patterns with your client. Good positioning helps clients to become more functional and improves the quality of their movement. Comfort and safety are maximized, and the person is easier to care for.

Fine Motor Tasks

Fine motor tasks are activities that involve using the hands and arms to reach, grasp, or release an object. Such tasks require coordinating vision with arm and hand movements so the person can reach accurately for an object and explore it with vision and touch.

Appropriate positioning can promote more controlled fine motor movements or more successful attempts at movement. If the individual uses a wheelchair or corner chair, encourage the person to rest the elbows on the tray to enhance arm and hand movements and give shoulder support. In addition to allowing greater arm and hand movements, this improves head and neck control. Using the tray during feeding helps individuals self-feed and improves head and neck control in individuals who require help with feeding. The client who requires staff assistance with feeding must always be in an upright position in a chair that provides appropriate support and positioning. (Refer to chapter 7 for information on feeding positions.)

If the client's movements are influenced by abnormal reflexes, fine motor tasks such as reaching for objects may be easier in an alternative position such as sidelying. In sidelying, the effect of abnormal reflexes on movement is minimized because the head is in midline and slightly forward. Position objects so the person can look slightly down and forward. This forward-bending head position will decrease the influence of abnormal reflex patterns. Extending the client's head behind the body will cause more straightening of the arms, legs, and back (extension), which will make attempts at fine motor tasks more difficult.

Activities of Daily Living

Activities of daily living (ADLs) refer to tasks that a person completes for self-care, such as feeding, dressing, hygiene, and housekeeping chores. Good positioning during such activities can maximize a client's ability to actively participate in them. Appropriate positioning may allow the person to assist with tasks such as brushing the teeth or self-feeding (finger feeding). If a client has difficulty completing an activity, try it in another position. If, for example, some of your clients show an interest in reaching down to help pull up their socks, you may try the following: Seat yourself behind the client, with both of you straddling a bolster. Or try the activity in sidelying or with the client in a feeder chair that is positioned securely on the floor. Look for movement patterns that are easier in particular positions—different tasks may require different positions.

Positioning and Communication

The effect of positioning upon both verbal and nonverbal communication should not be overlooked or underestimated. Communication is a daily interactive process. Proper positioning aids communication in several ways. For sound production, the client must be aligned to allow for a good breathing pattern. The airway needs to be straight from the rib cage to the mouth, and a stable posture improves the function of the muscles of sound production. If the individual is to point to, look at, touch, or attend to some kind of communicative device, keep in mind the type of movement needed and how the device should be placed for easiest access (see chapter 11 on switch mechanisms).

Most probably, the person you are working with does not produce words or many sounds. Communication is no less important for this person. Other responses such as body movement, facial expression, gestures, and eye contact can be first attempts at communication. Be a good observer and watch for different responses. Often you will see different communication responses in various positions.

Specific Guidelines for Positioning

Wheelchair

The wheelchair is used for transport, feeding, and fine motor and communication activities. Many models are available from several different companies. Adaptations can be added to support the head, shoulder girdle, and trunk. Some chairs have wedges that fit between the knees to keep them apart and in line with the hips. Special seats can be added to decrease the influence of abnormal tone, and footrests, armrests, and trays can be modified to fit the needs of the individual client. Plastic inserts can be custom molded to fit the individual. Some chairs convert to car seats; most can be secured into vans for transport.

Common problems encountered

1. *Posturing into extension.* This usually occurs with increased muscle tone. It is important to keep the hips flexed and pulled back in the chair. The seat belt should be snug across the hips and the foot straps fastened to stabilize the feet.

2. *Sliding forward in the chair with the back rounded and the knees too far apart.* This usually occurs with decreased muscle tone. To avoid this, make sure the seat belt is securely fastened across the hips. A towel roll can be placed on the outside of each thigh to keep the knees closer together.

3. *Asymmetry.* Asymmetry occurs with improper alignment of one part or several parts of the body. Often you will notice that the back curves to the side or that the knees or hips are not level. When this problem occurs, trunk supports are often added to keep the back straight. Make sure the hips are centered in the chair with the seat belt across the top of both hips.

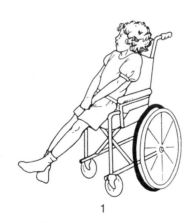

1

Posturing into extension

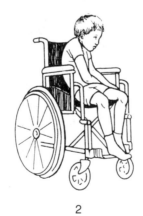

2

Poor posture seen with hypotonia

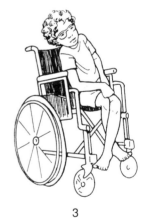

3

Asymmetrical posture

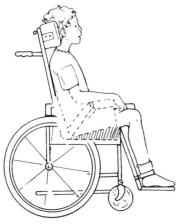

Proper positioning in a wheelchair

Proper positioning in a wheelchair

The back should be straight against the chair, with the knees slightly higher than the hips if the seat is wedged. Tighten the seat belt snugly to pull the hips back into the chair. Position the feet flat on the footrest, with the toes pointing straight ahead. Fasten the foot straps securely. The head should be at midline with the face straight ahead and centered in the head support. Make sure the shoulders, hips, and knees are all level. If the individual is properly seated following these guidelines, the listed problems should not occur.

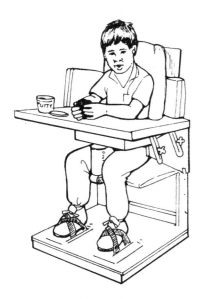

Proper positioning in a corner chair

Corner Chair

Corner chairs are often used for fine motor or visual activities or for feeding. They work well with clients who are unable to sit independently. Many come with detachable trays. Corner chairs are designed to keep the shoulders and arms forward and the head in midline.

Proper positioning in a corner chair

The seat, tray, and back heights need to be adjusted to the size of the client. The top of the chair should be level with the top of the head, and the tray should be at elbow height. Make sure the seat belt is securely fastened. Position the hips, knees, and ankles at 90-degree angles. If the back of the chair is too low, the head and neck can extend backward into an abnormal position. If the tray is too low, the client may fall forward and have difficulty holding up the head.

Sidelyer

The sidelyer is used to attain symmetry and to make it easier for the hands to function at the middle of the body. It is helpful with clients who have poor head control or who have difficulty holding objects in an upright position. The sidelyer positions the client so that the face and hands are in optimal alignment for using the hands and eyes together.

Proper positioning in a sidelyer

The back should be flat or slightly rounded against the frame of the side-lyer with the head in midline and slightly forward. Bring the shoulders forward and the hands together. Bend the hips and knees and put a small pillow between the legs. If the legs are not properly positioned, they will tend to move in abnormal spastic patterns, which will then cause abnormal movements to occur in the head and upper body.

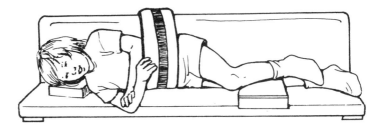

Proper positioning in a sidelyer

Standing Frame

The standing frame is used with clients who cannot stand alone but who need the experience of being in an upright position. The standing position is important especially for older children and adults. It is socially beneficial for them to view their surroundings from an age-appropriate height. The upright weight-bearing position is also beneficial for the proper growth of the hip joint. Standing frames often come with removable trays so they can be used during hand activities. Some of them can stand next to a counter top, and most of them can be angled for clients who cannot tolerate standing completely upright.

Proper positioning in a standing frame

The top of the frame should end two inches below the client's armpit, leaving the hands free for fine motor activities. If the frame comes too close to the armpit, the client will tend to "hang" on the frame rather than taking weight on the legs. Make sure the back is straight and the head at midline. If the person doesn't bear weight equally on both legs, the back can curve to the side, creating abnormal alignment. Position the knees slightly apart and straighten them as much as possible. The feet should point straight ahead and be flat on the footrest. Many clients have difficulty completely straightening the hips, so most standing frames come with a thick strap that supports the hips. Make sure this strap is snugly fastened.

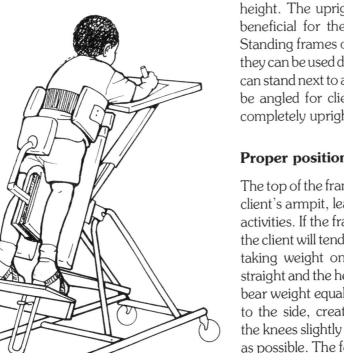

Proper positioning in a standing frame

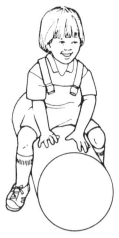

Proper positioning on a bolster

Bolsters and Wedges

Bolsters and wedges are pieces of equipment to be used only when you are directly supervising a client.

Bolsters

Bolsters are useful in helping clients to improve their balance in the sitting position. Sit behind the client with both of you straddling the bolster. Make sure the client's feet are flat on the floor and the knees are directly in line with the hips. The back should be straight, the head at midline, and the shoulders forward. Support the client's back with your body. Put your hands on top of the client's knees to control the position of the legs. Don't allow the knees to come together. Then slowly roll the bolster from side to side.

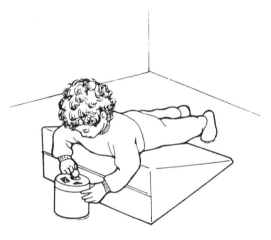

Proper positioning on a wedge

Wedges

Use a wedge for working on raising the head and reaching in stomach lying. The STNR and the tonic reflex make it difficult for many clients to lift the head while lying on the stomach supported on bent elbows. The wedge makes it easier for the client to overcome the effects of these abnormal reflexes. Lay the client on the wedge with the shoulders slightly beyond the edge of the wedge. The legs should be separated. Sit in front of the client, and bring the elbows and shoulders forward to bear weight. Encourage head lifting by calling the person or by offering an object to reach for. If the client cannot reach independently, assist with the motion. Clients left unsupervised on a wedge tend to collapse over the edge, and their head falls down. Don't use the wedge to position clients if you aren't going to be working with them.

Positioning considerations are also important for clients who use regular furniture. Make sure the chair is high enough so that the client is able to place both feet flat on the floor. If the chair is too high, a small stool can be placed under the feet. The feet can then help to stabilize the rest of the body. The chair should be close enough to the table for easy reaching, and the seat needs to be high enough for the client to place the elbows on the table. In an upholstered chair, rolled towels can be used to stabilize the upper body.

When an individual is capable of little voluntary movement, positioning during sleep is important. Sleeping positions can be changed during the night from back lying to the right or left sides. In sidelying, putting a pillow between the legs to keep them slightly apart is a good idea. This will decrease the effects of abnormal tone and reflexive responses. Some clients are comfortable hugging a pillow in the sidelying position. In back lying, the tonic reflex can be diminished by keeping the head forward on a pillow and by putting a pillow under the knees. Pillows also can be placed slightly behind the shoulders to keep them forward. Stomach lying is often uncomfortable for individuals with spasticity and strong reflexes.

Adaptive Equipment Checklist

Name:_____ Age:_____

Date: _____ Primary Caregiver: _____

Check off equipment used by this individual.

   _____ wheelchair   _____ standing frame

   _____ corner chair   _____ bolster

   _____ feeder seat   _____ wedge

   _____ sidelyer

As you use this equipment, refer to the following guidelines. If you cannot achieve these positions, you may need to modify the equipment, or the equipment may not be appropriate for this individual.

Wheelchair

_____ 1. Is the back straight, and are the knees and hips level?

_____ 2. Are the hips pulled back into the chair?

_____ 3. Are the shoulders level and the head at midline?

Corner Chair/Feeder Seat

_____ 1. Is the chair back properly adjusted to entirely support the back of the head?

_____ 2. Are the hips, knees, and ankles bent at 90-degree angles?

_____ 3. Is the tray adjusted to elbow height?

Standing Frame

_____ 1. Are the feet, back, and knees straight?

_____ 2. Are the arms free to reach?

_____ 3. Is the client strapped in for safety?

Sidelyer

_____ 1. Is the head at midline?

_____ 2. Are the shoulders forward and the hands together?

_____ 3. Are the knees separated?

Concerns found: _____

_____

_____

Action taken: _____

_____

_____

7
Feeding and Oral-Motor Concerns

Why are feeding guidelines and recommendations important?

Each one of us experiences the mealtime routine from the day we are born. It should be an enjoyable time that is anticipated with pleasure. Feeding is one of the first interactions that is mutually satisfying for both the baby and the caregiver. How one responds to the meal and the process of eating often sets the tone for other interactions throughout the day. The quantity and types of foods we eat obviously influence our health. Eating affects our moods, can alter our behavior, and is life sustaining. It can also become a measure of success for the caregiver. What mother doesn't feel a sense of accomplishment when, after a meal, all the plates are licked clean? Frequently, when a baby or child doesn't eat well, the care provider feels like a failure at something that is supposed to be very easy. All too often one's worth is measured by the quantity of food consumed. A sense of failure can easily be turned inward when the child eats meagerly or refuses to eat altogether.

These are some important considerations to be aware of before addressing the specific feeding difficulties often associated with a severe handicap. Recognizing the social importance of eating can, we hope, prevent you from feeling that you have failed when clients don't eat the way you think they should. The notion that more is better is not necessarily true and, all too frequently, is not in one's best interest. The method of feeding is just as important as the number of calories consumed. The pleasure and enjoyment most of us associate with a good meal is frequently not experienced by the person with severe disabilities. Instead, due to physical limitations, mealtime for such a person means being a nonparticipating recipient, and it is a time of coughing, choking, and discomfort. Both the individual and the care provider are more likely to experience anxiety and frustration than pleasure. Feeding is often a one-way process, with the provider in complete control.

Hence, the challenge is to do everything possible to get rid of the "road blocks" and provide a pleasurable eating experience that is environmentally appealing, nutritionally sound, and safe, while using to the fullest each person's individual skills and encouraging an active two-way interaction. It's no fun to be a passive recipient with no role in the activity!

What are the goals of feeding guidelines?

1. To encourage the best and safest use of oral skills during eating and drinking

2. To present a variety of foods in a safe manner while encouraging the person to use existing feeding skills and, ultimately, to develop more advanced skills

3. To give the individual an opportunity to be independent and to assist with eating

4. To complete meals within a reasonable length of time

5. To achieve a neater, more socially acceptable eating pattern

6. To ensure that active, intentional communication is occurring between the individual and the caregiver.

Reducing Feeding Problems

These factors will help make feeding more successful and enjoyable:

Positioning

Positioning can be crucial to the individual's ability to self-feed and to your ability to assist the person with eating. Good positioning is beneficial in (a) decreasing high muscle tone, (b) supporting low muscle tone, (c) reducing the influence of abnormal reflexes, (d) promoting social interaction, (e) decreasing the client's risk of choking (aspiration), and (f) making the experience more enjoyable for all concerned. Your feedback regarding how the individual responds in different positions during mealtimes can be extremely valuable to the consulting therapists. Similarly, consistent follow-through with positioning recommendations is very important so the benefits of treatment can be assessed.

Texture of foods and liquids

Texture refers to the consistency of a food or liquid. For example, water is the thinnest consistency of liquid that we consume. Different textures require different mouth movements in order to safely move the food to the back of the mouth and swallow it. Simply because all of a child's baby teeth are present does not mean the child can safely tolerate a regular diet consistency, such as a plate of vegetables, french fries, and a hamburger. Your observations of how well the person tolerates different food items coupled with an *oral-motor assessment* completed by either the speech-language pathologist or the occupational therapist will indicate the best food and liquid textures for each person.

Oral treatment

Oral treatment means giving some type of assistance to the mouth, face, or jaw area to make eating safer and easier. The purpose is to help the person feel the sensations of a normal movement pattern. This "feeling" may be new and strange to someone who is accustomed only to abnormal reflexive movements. Because the person is accustomed to old habits and abnormal patterns, oral treatment may be met with anxiety, fear, and resistance. Consistent and correct use of these techniques will help the person learn a better and safer way to eat or drink.

There are many types of oral treatment, and your consulting professional can help you determine which is most suitable for each individual's needs. Some examples of oral treatment that may be used include:

> *Oral stimulation.* These techniques can be used before feeding or in place of oral feeding for the client who is tube fed. Before feeding, the emphasis may be to decrease high sensitivity, to decrease abnormal patterns, or to increase muscle tone. During tube feedings, oral stimulation is important to promote oral functions and to provide a pleasurable experience for the individual. A specific example would be massaging a client's cheeks in a circular motion with one or two fingers.

> *External positioning.* External positioning keeps the neck from hyperextending (leaning way back) during swallowing. This type of positioning is done using a wheelchair or other seating device.

> *Jaw control.* Jaw control is a specific technique to assist a client with poor jaw movements. This technique involves placing your index finger under a client's lip and your middle finger under the chin to help with jaw movements during eating and drinking. The consulting occupational therapist and/or speech-language pathologist will determine whether this technique would benefit a particular individual.

Adaptive equipment

Adaptive equipment can be used by the client or the caretaker to make oral feeding or stimulation safer and easier. Equipment ranges from specialized utensils and plates to special cups and nonslip materials. As you assist an individual to eat, your observations of cup or utensil use can be valuable information for the professional working with you.

Feeding Guidelines: Some Do's and Don'ts

Do	*Don't*
1. Approach with a greeting, something to signal that a move or change in action is going to occur.	Cause a startle response.
2. Know how to position each person appropriately for a meal. Know what adaptive equipment to use and how to use it before moving the person.	Put yourself or the client at risk for injury.
3. Know how to manage the transfer in the best and safest way. Know your limitations and when and how to use a two- or three-person lift.	Consider carrying the client around while trying to locate the necessary equipment.
4. Use necessary safety straps.	Put the client at risk.
5. Use prescribed adaptive feeding equipment and communication aids, such as switches, pictures, communication boards.	Run in and out of the area to gather the equipment.
6. Position yourself optimally for eye contact, conversation, and use of prescribed therapy techniques. Try to sit directly in front of the person.	Assume a hovering position over the person.
7. Complete recommended oral stimulation prior to introducing the meal.	Attempt oral stimulation if you have not been trained in the procedure or if you do not know what you are trying to accomplish.
8. Approach with the spoon from below the chin up to the mouth.	Bring the spoon from eye level or above down toward the mouth.
9. Encourage a midline head position with a slight chin tuck.	Allow the head to tip backwards when receiving food or drink.
10. Bring the spoon straight out of the mouth, encouraging upper lip movement to remove food from the spoon.	Scrape the spoon on the teeth.
11. Make sure the food and liquid are the proper texture (such as puréed or bite size) and temperature.	Alter food or liquid texture without approval from a therapist.

Feeding Guidelines: Some Do's and Don'ts (continued)

Do	*Don't*
12. Present small amounts on the spoon.	Give many spoonfuls rapidly without allowing the person to swallow safely.
13. Use recommended oral therapy techniques (such as jaw control).	Use oral techniques without training.
14. Use a slow pace regardless of the person's eating skills.	Rush the meal.
15. Remember to speak to the person in a pleasant conversational tone.	Yell at the person to "swallow!"
16. Press the spoon down gently yet firmly on the middle part of the front third of the tongue.	Continue to give food or liquid if the person begins choking, coughing, or gagging.
17. Release a bite reflex through massaging the cheeks, pushing up on the chin, or rubbing the outside of the gums.	Yell, "Let go!" or pull on the spoon in order to get a release.
18. Be aware that some people respond adversely to hot or cold foods.	Force your preferences or dislikes on the person you are feeding.
19. Give small sips of liquids throughout the meal.	Force an entire cup of fluid down rapidly at the beginning or end of the meal.
20. Place the cup on the lower lip, making sure the tongue is under the cup.	Flood the person's mouth with liquid.
21. Use a warm or lukewarm cloth for cleansing the face and hands. Try to blot just one time across the mouth and chin, using moderate pressure on the skin, then wiping up off the face.	Wipe the mouth with a cloth after every spoonful, or use the spoon to scrape food off the face repeatedly.
22. Expect the person's face (and hands) to get somewhat messy during the meal.	Wipe the face repeatedly; this can be too stimulating.
23. Speak in a conversational tone about what you're doing and other events.	Be mechanical and silent!
24. Allow the person the opportunity to signal for more or to refuse food.	Anticipate every movement and need.

General Environmental Suggestions and Guidelines

Try to do everything possible to ensure a pleasurable eating experience, beginning with the environment. The following checklist provides help with guidelines to ensure a pleasant atmosphere.

Environment

_____ Is the atmosphere relaxing, and does it appear comfortable?

_____ Is the appearance of the room appealing?

_____ Is the area clean?

_____ Is the room temperature comfortable?

_____ Is the lighting too dark or too bright?

_____ Is the television off?

_____ Can background music be tolerated?

_____ Is the radio or stereo too loud?

_____ Are outside disruptions or interruptions being kept to a minimum?

Interaction

_____ Is there an appropriate activity for the individual to participate in while waiting for the meal or following the meal, when your attention is directed elsewhere?

_____ Are people seated so they have the opportunity to interact with each other?

_____ Is there enough space to accommodate needed seating arrangements?

_____ Can adapted or regular dining room chairs be used rather than wheelchairs?

_____ Can you sit at eye level and interact with the clients rather than hovering above them?

_____ Can you speak to the clients in a normal conversational voice and be heard?

_____ Are individuals dressed and groomed appropriately for the meal?

_____ Is there a method for handling disruptive behavior that causes the least possible amount of distraction to other eaters?

_____ Are the individuals actively involved in the mealtime process and cleanup to the greatest extent possible?

_____ Does each person receive some type of individualized attention?

Equipment

_____ Is adaptive equipment being used as prescribed? This includes cups, utensils, dishes, and lap trays, as well as positioning equipment.

_____ Are switches or communication aids being used?

Food Texture and Appearance

_____ Does the food look and smell appealing?

_____ Is the correct food texture being presented?

_____ If the meal is puréed, can you tell that there are separate foods, rather than everything being all mixed together?

_____ Are liquids presented intermittently throughout the meal, rather than all at once at the end of the meal?

Medication

_____ Do medical procedures interfere with the meal?

_____ Are medications in plain view; are they threatening?

_____ Are designated techniques being followed for administering medications (for example, correct positioning or use of an adaptive spoon)?

Positioning

Correct positioning during oral feeding is one of the most important areas of care. Proper positioning can (1) promote better oral function and better swallowing, (2) lessen the risk of accidentally getting liquid and food into the lungs (*aspiration*), (3) provide better social and interactive contact, and (4) allow for more self-feeding by the client. Good positioning during feeding can lessen the influence of abnormal reflex patterns, which may improve feeding.

The majority of clients should be sitting in a wheelchair or well supported in adaptive seating for feeding. As discussed in chapter 6, some general guidelines should be followed when positioning an individual for meals or presenting anything by mouth.

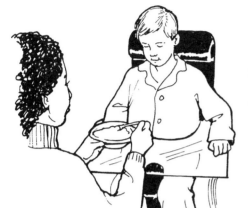

In good feeding position, the person should have a slight chin tuck, and the arms should be supported on a wheelchair tray or table.

1. The client's hips should be pulled back into the chair, with the knees and hips bent and level, the back straight, and the feet supported.

2. The shoulders should be level and the head at midline.

3. The individual's head and neck should be slightly bent forward so the chin is slightly tucked. Can you assist the client into a chin tuck easily?

   During feeding, the client's head should be slightly flexed forward to decrease the effect of abnormal reflexes and make swallowing easier. Have you ever tried swallowing either while lying down or with your head tilted back? Try it—and you will see how much easier it is with the chin tucked.

4. The person's arms and elbows should be supported on a table or tray.

Head and neck control and mouth movements will be better if the client's arms are supported on a table or wheelchair tray. This support adds stability through the shoulders, helps with head and neck control, and makes using the arms and hands easier. This positioning also helps with body alignment and keeping the shoulders level.

Your positioning can also influence the oral function of the person you are feeding or assisting. Try to sit directly in front of a person you are spoon feeding, at or slightly below eye level.

This will encourage the client to keep the head bent slightly forward and in midline. Approach the client with the spoon below eye level, telling the person as you start your approach that you are giving another "bite" or spoonful. If the client is visually impaired, verbal and tactile cues are especially important.

Another consideration is your comfort during feeding or oral stimulation activities. Some of these techniques require you to stand next to the client for extended periods. It is a good idea to elevate one foot on a low surface (such as a block or step) to decrease back stress. This will help both you and the client to be relaxed and comfortable.

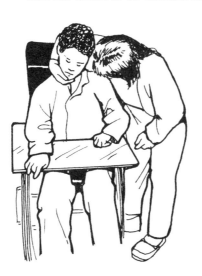

The caregiver is incorrectly positioned in a stressful and uncomfortable posture.

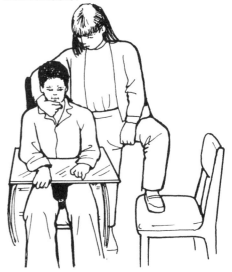

Try to assume feeding positions that are comfortable for both you and the client.

Other feeding positions may be recommended by the therapy team. If this is the case, please refer to those professionals for specific positioning recommendations.

Swallowing Function and Dysfunction

Swallowing refers to the action of transporting food or liquid from the mouth to the stomach. Swallowing is an action most people take for granted. For most of us it occurs routinely without much thought or effort—until something such as an earache or a sore throat interferes with the process. For people with a neurological or motor disorder, however, swallowing can be a difficult and effortful process.

Swallowing is a highly complex process that seems to involve both involuntary and voluntary movements. Once the food or liquid reaches a certain point in the back of the mouth, a swallow is triggered automatically. On the other hand, you can swallow without having any food or liquid in your mouth. This swallowing is voluntary. Swallowing actually takes place in three stages:

1. *Oral stage.* During the oral stage food is moved around, chewed, or held within the mouth and prepared to be moved to the back of the mouth.

2. *Pharyngeal stage.* The pharyngeal stage begins when the food passes over the back of the tongue in transit to the esophagus (the tube that leads to the stomach).

3. *Esophageal stage.* During the esophageal stage, food enters the stomach and undergoes the initial digestive process.

During a swallow a number of coordinated changes occur in the muscles and structures of the throat area that allow the food or liquid to be transported to the correct destination. Any dysfunction at any stage of the swallowing process can adversely affect one's ability to eat. The primary concern in a swallowing difficulty is the potential for *aspiration.* In aspiration, a foreign body (such as body secretions, food, or liquid) is inhaled into the lungs rather than going into the stomach. Aspiration can lead to choking or difficulty breathing and contribute to poor health, illness, and even death.

In addition to having poor oral skills, the person may have a swallowing disorder. The only way to tell for certain that a swallowing disorder does exist is through *radiographic* (X-ray) study. The technique is called *fluoroscopy,* which is a radiographic technique permitting observation of movement. Rather than taking a still X-ray, a moving X-ray is filmed while the individual eats a barium-coated food item or drinks a barium mixture in an upright posture. The swallowing movement can be viewed on a monitor. This procedure is called a *modified barium swallow* study. Information obtained in this way will indicate types of oral treatment to be used and whether or not eating by mouth is safe. Aspiration is discovered frequently, even when the individual does not cough, choke, or give any clue that food is going into the lungs. This is called *silent aspiration.*

Recommendations for Administration of Medications

Because we think of taking medications by mouth as being different from eating a snack or a meal, it's easy to forget about feeding guidelines. It is very important, however, to follow these guidelines when giving medication as well.

Because medications usually have a telltale smell and taste, they may be accepted more easily when they are disguised in a food item. Just as foods or liquids may need to have certain consistencies, so, too, may medications. For example, liquid medications are easier to mix in yogurt or pudding than are solid pills. Likewise a pill that can be crushed can be mixed more easily than a whole tablet. If an individual is having difficulty taking medication, check with your medical professional regarding whether the medicine can be administered in an alternative form or mixed with food.

The bottom line is getting the medication safely into the person's system. A pill that gets into the lungs rather than the stomach does no good and, moreover, puts the person at risk for further health problems. You have a responsibility not only to administer medication, but to present it safely.

Guidelines for Medication Presentation

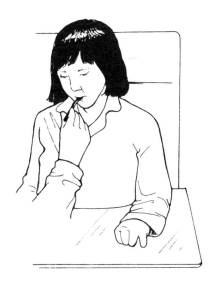

Remember to follow the same guidelines when giving medications as you do for feeding.

1. The individual must be upright. Simply because the medication can be swallowed in only one or two swallows, you cannot dispense with good positioning. At a minimum, the upper trunk must be elevated. The head needs to be upright and at midline, with a slight chin tuck. Swallowing will be easier if the hips are in an "L" position and the legs are bent at the knees and well supported.

2. If allowable, mix the medicine with a food or liquid of a consistency the person can tolerate. Medicine is usually better accepted if it can be presented with a meal.

3. Use the adaptive equipment that has been specified for the individual. If a person uses a coated spoon to eat, then the medication also should be presented using a coated spoon. Place the spoon in the middle of the tongue, on the front third portion. Press downward until the tongue starts to hump back. Remove the spoon straight out of the mouth, taking care not to scrape it on the teeth.

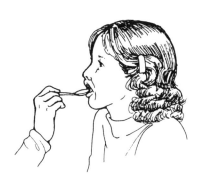

Present the medication on the spoon, pushing gently but firmly down and back on the first third of the tongue.

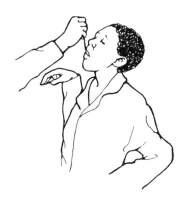

Do not scrape the medicine off the spoon, as this may cause the person's head to tilt back.

4. Tell the person what you are doing. You don't need to say, "John, here comes your big ugly pill," but rather, "John, here is a spoonful of applesauce," or "John, it's time to take a drink of juice."

5. Use facilitation techniques, if necessary, to help the person swallow. *Do not ever block the airway*—for example by plugging the person's nose. If you have difficulty getting the mouth open or closed, the occupational therapist or speech-language pathologist may be able to show you helpful techniques. Do not yell at the person to "swallow!"

6. Be considerate. If the medicine is not disguised, give a taste of liquid or a pleasurable food item to help get rid of the taste of the medicine.

Overview of Feeding Problems

The problems discussed in this section are often seen in individuals with developmental disabilities. However, just as you are an individual with unique strengths and weaknesses, so too are people with neurological disorders. Some will have normal oral-motor function; others will have a variety of problems that may interfere with feeding, drinking, swallowing, or speech. Some patterns or groups of difficulties can occur together. The people you work with may or may not have the following problems. Please ask a therapist to discuss with you what oral-motor (feeding) difficulties your clients show and specific treatment approaches to use with them.

Reflexive Problems

Abnormal reflexes (see chapter 4) can also interfere with feeding. A reflex is a consistent response to a particular touch or position. Remember that reflexes *cannot* be controlled by the individual. Specific examples include these:

Tonic bite reflex

Some clients clamp the jaw closed when anything (such as a spoon, finger, or toothbrush) is placed on the teeth. It is important to have a therapist assess all clients for oral reflexes. If the person has a bite reflex you don't know about, you could be injured by the person biting down on your finger during feeding, or the client could be injured by biting down on a hard object. For safety, never use a glass container for drinking or metal utensils for feeding. Either of these may injure the mouth if the client does have a bite reflex. For obvious reasons, never stick your fingers in the person's mouth, unless you have been shown specific techniques.

Treatment suggestions for a tonic bite reflex

1. Appropriate positioning will reduce muscle tone and may modify the frequency and intensity of this reflex.

2. If the person has bitten down on an object (such as a spoon), you can try the following:

   - Massage the cheeks by making circular movements with one of two of your fingers on both cheeks.
   - Massage the outer gums with one finger; start at the middle of the front teeth and rub firmly toward the back of the mouth two or three times on each side.
   - Push up gently but firmly on the chin. (You may elicit a reverse reaction that causes the person to open the mouth.)

Remember: Never try to pull the object out of the mouth by force. You may hurt the person or loosen teeth!

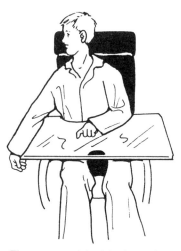

The asymmetrical tonic reflex (ATNR) can influence muscle tone on both sides of the body and change movements the person is attempting.

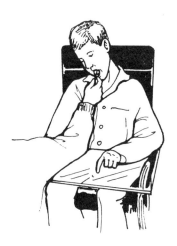

If an individual is influenced by the ATNR, position the head in the center of the body and present food at midline.

Asymmetrical tonic neck reflex (ATNR)

This reflex, described in chapter 4, may also have an influence on feeding. It may not only cause the head to turn to one side, but may also cause changes in muscle tone on both sides of the body. The ATNR, if strong and elicited during a swallow, may also affect the person's swallowing pattern. For a person who is self-feeding, the ATNR can substantially interfere with attempts to bring food to the mouth. The reflex may cause the head to turn as the person bends the elbow to bring a spoon or cup to the mouth.

Treatment suggestions for ATNR

1. Positioning is the key. If you are feeding an individual, sit in front of the person and help to keep the head in midline.

2. Present food at midline and encourage the person to look straight ahead.

3. If you are using a wheelchair tray or table, position the person's arms on the tray in front of the body. If the person is self-feeding, set up as much of the meal as possible in the middle of the tray or table. Position utensils so the person's attention and head position stay at midline.

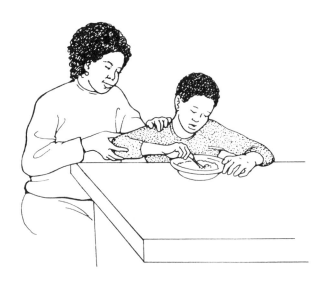

Assisting a client to self-feed.
Note that the bowl is in midline to prevent the ATNR.

Problem Areas

Head and neck tipped back

Clients with either too much muscle tone (hypertonia) or too little muscle tone (hypotonia) may have poor head and neck control. These individuals often tip the head back into hyperextension to stabilize it while sitting. This position has been called the *bird feeding* position. Although this position may appear to help feeding, it *does not!* Eating or drinking with the head tilted back greatly increases the risk that the food or drink will be aspirated (taken into the lungs). This position may also result in poor lip, tongue, and jaw movements.

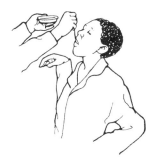

Example of bird feeding. This is *not* a good feeding position.

Treatment suggestions for bird feeding

1. Ask the advice of your feeding therapist.

2. Reposition the client in the chair, making sure the person hasn't slipped so that the hips are straight and resting on the front of the chair. Keeping the hips back and bent will help to reduce high muscle tone. For feeding, keep the individual as upright as possible.

3. Do not try pressing on the back of the head to force it forward. Trying to push a person into a position by force usually only increases the strength of the movement in the opposite direction. Thus, pushing the head forward may cause greater neck extension. Try positioning the head from above by gently but firmly applying pressure downward and forward.

4. Use other techniques your therapist may have shown you (such as jaw control) to improve head and neck position during feeding.

5. Try to offer the food or drink at or below eye level, so the person is not inclined to look up or tip the head back.

6. Place the person's arms forward on the wheelchair tray or a table.

7. The feeding therapists may suggest alternative feeding positions for a client (especially a child) if neck hyperextension cannot be corrected in a seated position. If so, please follow the therapists' recommendations.

Tongue thrusting

Tongue thrusting may occur if an individual has either too little or too much muscle tone. The tongue typically appears to be pushing out strongly when the person tries to eat or drink. Tongue thrusting is a strong reaction that *cannot* be controlled by the client. It can sometimes be seen with *suckling,* which is the backward and forward motion of the tongue that moves food back in the mouth for swallowing.

Treatment suggestions for tongue thrusting

1. Position the client appropriately in a wheelchair or other appropriate seating arrangement.

2. As you present a spoonful of food—with a coated spoon—press down and back gently but firmly on the front third of the tongue.

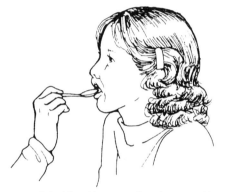

Present a spoonful of food by pressing down and back firmly
but gently on the first third of the tongue.

3. Sweet, sugary foods may increase suckling and tongue thrust. You may want to avoid sugary foods because they also increase saliva and dental decay.

4. With cup drinking, place the cup on the lower lip, with the tongue in the mouth and under the cup. Using a cut-out cup may help you to control cup placement and regulate the amount of liquid given by allowing you to see how much liquid you are giving.

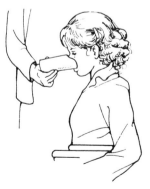

Place a cut-out cup on the person's lower lip,
with the tongue under the cup to help with drinking.

Poor lip closure

A person needs to be able to bring the lips together in order to take food off a spoon, keep food or liquid in the mouth, and drink without most of the liquid dribbling out. Poor lip control can be related to decreased muscle tone, in which the client generally has an *open mouth* posture, or tight muscle tone, in which the lips are *retracted* (pulled back).

Treatment suggestions for poor lip closure

1. A slight chin tuck during feeding and drinking will often facilitate lip closure.

2. As you present the spoon, push down gently but firmly on the client's tongue, and then wait patiently for the individual to try to bring the upper lip down. Please *do not* scrape food off the spoon using the client's upper teeth. Doing so promotes neck hyperextension and poor feeding habits.

3. After the client takes a bite, you can support the lower lip and jaw with one hand as shown to keep the food from dribbling out of the client's mouth.

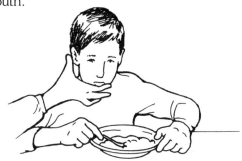

Assisting with lip closure for a client who is self-feeding.

4. With cup drinking, you may need to assist with upper or lower lip closure (not both) on the cup. Support the upper or lower lip with your finger during drinking. Take away your help as the individual develops independent lip closure.

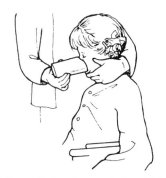

Assisting with lip closure during drinking

5. Specific techniques to improve lip closure may be part of a therapeutic feeding program. Please check with the relevant therapist(s).

Jaw opening or clamping

Excessive jaw opening or jaw clamping may be seen. Clamping may be involuntary and related to muscle tone or a tonic bite reflex. It could also be a behavioral response. This problem must, therefore, be evaluated by the treatment team so they can give you strategies for coping with it. Jaw opening (thrusting) may be related either to hypertonicity or to hypotonicity. A person with low muscle tone often has an open mouth position, in which the jaw is open and may be unstable. Chewing skills are often poor due to jaw instability and decreased muscle tone, with poor tongue movements. In individuals with high muscle tone, the excessive jaw opening usually is related to an extensor (straightening) pattern or thrust. Clients who have difficulty smoothly opening and closing the jaw also may show this pattern and are likely to have poor chewing skills. As they anticipate food or drink coming toward them, they open their jaws too widely, usually with neck hyperextension.

Treatment suggestions for jaw opening or clamping

1. Appropriate positioning is again essential. Provide trunk support for a client with low muscle tone—use a harness or wheelchair tray and seat belt. Secure the feet on footrests; support the head and neck as needed. Individuals with high muscle tone should be positioned with the hips and knees bent, the head at midline, and the chin slightly tucked to decrease abnormal tone and reflex influences.

2. Try to maintain a chin tuck during mealtime by presenting utensils below eye level.

3. Talk to the person throughout the meal. Telling a person with poor jaw control to anticipate a spoonful of food may help to prepare the person, resulting in a less abnormal response.

4. Your therapist may demonstrate additional jaw control techniques for certain clients.

There are additional problem areas that are not discussed in this chapter. Specific oral-motor difficulties require intervention programs designed by the therapy team. The treatment approaches discussed in this section are general and should be reviewed and supplemented by the therapist who is treating your clients.

Oral-Motor Sensitivity Problems

Individuals with disabilities may show mild to extreme responses to the sensory stimuli we experience every day—temperature, touch, texture (that is, rough versus smooth), sounds, smells, or amount of light. Your clients' responses to a sensory stimulus may not be what you would expect from a nonhandicapped person in the same situation. Or their responses may seem normal for a period of time, but after repeated sensory stimulation, they begin reacting to it.

In regard to oral-motor issues, clients with sensory sensitivities may react to touch, sound, or temperatures or textures of foods or liquids. Some of these problems also may have a behavioral component, but many persons genuinely do have problems with their sensory systems. Some key behaviors to look for will be discussed in the following section.

Temperature of foods and liquids

An individual may show a severe or mild reaction to foods that are either hot or cold. Typical responses are lip pursing or lip retraction (pulling the lips back tightly into a thin line), or refusal to eat or drink more. For an individual who is sensitive to food temperature, you may want to serve most foods at room temperature or just slightly warmed.

Textures of foods and liquids

Some clients react to foods with a coarser texture than a purée. Responses that typically indicate oral hypersensitivity include the following:

- Gagging
- Separating the food in the mouth using the tongue. Clients swallow what they can tolerate and spit out or dribble out what they cannot handle (generally the larger pieces).
- Refusing to eat or drink more
- Vomiting
- Holding foods in the mouth

A treatment program for this type of sensitivity should be developed by a trained therapist. Your contribution comes in behavior management, following treatment guidelines consistently, and using a gentle but firm approach.

Sensitivity to touch

Some individuals do not like being touched. This reaction may be localized inside or outside the client's mouth or be generalized to a person's entire body. Indicators of hypersensitivity to touch include the following:

- Attempts to move away from touch by head turning or body movement
- Increased irritability as you handle the client during the process of daily care

When assisting with personal care needs, keep in mind that clients who display some degree of sensitivity to being touched (*tactile defensiveness*) generally will tolerate firm pressure best. Light touch, such as patting or stroking, is usually irritating to a client with tactile defensiveness. Though people with normal sensation find patting or stroking pleasurable, to an individual with touch sensitivity it may feel the way you feel when the hair on your arm is lightly touched or fingernails are scratched across a chalkboard.

Auditory/visual sensitivities

Again, as we all have individual likes and dislikes, so does the individual with a neurological impairment. Often overlooked in caretaking is the environment of these clients and how their sensitivities are bombarded inadvertently. Some residents may show these signs in response to light or sound:

- Startles or tremors to loud music or noises
- Increased irritability
- Withdrawal behaviors
- Decreased interaction

By being conscious of light sources and sound levels you can avoid over-stimulating the client and encourage more interaction, both among clients and between clients and staff, and increase individual comfort levels. Watching for nonverbal cues can help you to determine whether sounds or lights are bothering clients. In a group situation, modifying light and noise levels may be difficult, but some changes are possible. Decrease fluorescent lighting or hang blinds in the windows to filter daylight. Lower the volume of radios, TVs, and stereos. Shut doors quietly or install hydraulic closing devices. (Gluing foam padding around the door frame where the door closes against it will prevent the door from slamming.) Though these suggestions may seem minimal, they may make daily living more comfortable for people who startle easily and for their caretakers.

Non-Oral Feeding Considerations

Oral stimulation is important to all of us, even before birth. Eating has many pleasures and benefits we take for granted. As human beings, we receive intense pleasure from tasting foods, smelling, and being touched. As we eat, we use coordinated movements of our tongues, lips, and teeth. As we produce saliva, we coordinate a swallow. We usually interact with others, talking and listening as we eat. If it is necessary for a client to receive non-oral feedings, oral stimulation remains extremely important, as does how and when non-oral feedings occur. In this section, some of these issues will be addressed.

Some individuals with severe motor handicaps or poor oral-motor skills and swallowing patterns may receive nourishment through other means than by mouth. The two most common non-oral feeding methods are by tube feeding: A *nasogastric tube* (or NG tube) goes into the nose and down the esophagus into the stomach. A *gastrostomy* tube goes directly into the stomach. Tube feedings are usually started by a physician because of the following conditions:

1. Poor swallowing or risk of aspiration of food or liquid into the client's lungs

2. Structural problems that could make it difficult for the person to eat effectively

3. Increased vomiting or gastro-esophageal reflux; *reflux* occurs when fluids from the stomach back up into the esophagus and may cause aspiration.

Determining that a person would benefit from non-oral feedings does not imply a failure on the part of the client or the staff. Tube feedings can be a short-term or long-term means to provide life-sustaining nutrition.

Important Guidelines for Tube Feeding

1. Continue to provide oral stimulation, as recommended by the therapy team. Oral stimulation should be done during or before non-oral feedings, if possible.

2. Tube feedings should be "normalized" to regular feeding times. This encourages socialization during meals.

3. Positioning of the client continues to be important, both for the individual's comfort and for ease of tube feeding. The client should be as upright as feasible to allow interaction with others and to decrease reflux. (Reflux is the upward movement of the stomach's contents into the esophagus.)

4. If the non-oral feeding is not scheduled at mealtime, try to include social interaction in the feeding time. Isolating the individual perpetuates the perception that this form of feeding is very different from oral feeding and is likely to affect the person's self-esteem. Even though the client receives nourishment through a tube, the feeding is the individual's mealtime and should be made as pleasant as possible.

Adaptive Equipment

Some individuals with special needs benefit from using adaptive equipment during meals. To help you in identifying and properly using equipment, you will find on the following pages illustrations of selected equipment and reasons to use each piece.

Plate and Bowl Options

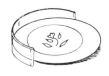

Plate guard

A plate guard builds up one side of a plate so food can be scooped against it.

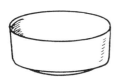

High-sided plate

All sides of a *high-sided plate* are built up to help in scooping food against the sides or keeping food on the plate.

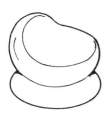

Scooper bowl

A *scooper bowl or plate* is used mainly for children. Again, one side is built up, and there is a suction base to decrease slippage.

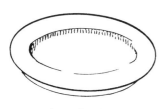

Inner lip plate

An *inner lip plate* has a built-in lip around the edge to aid in scooping food; it is generally used by adolescents or adults.

Utensils

Built-up handles can be placed or ordered on spoons, knives, or forks to allow a better gripping surface.

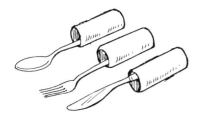

Built-up handles on utensils can give clients a better grasp.

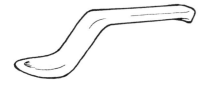

A universal cuff helps the person maintain grasp on a utensil.

A *universal cuff* is used to help a person maintain grasp on a utensil. The handle of the utensil slides into a pocket on the cuff. The cuff can then be strapped to the client's hand. The utensil is positioned as it would normally be held: the pocket (handle) fits in the palm of the hand, with the utensil coming out of the thumb side; the strap comes over the top of the person's hand, behind the knuckles.

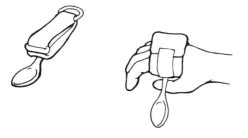

Nonmetal utensils

Nonmetal utensils are often recommended for clients with feeding problems. Several types of spoons and forks are commercially available. A second option is rubber-coated or plastic-coated utensils, which have a thin layer of material over the bowl of the spoon.

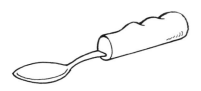

Weighted utensils

Weighted utensils have heavy handles to assist clients who have a tremor or a need for a heavier utensil.

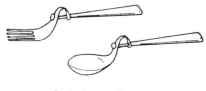

Swivel utensils

Swivel utensils are useful for clients with limited wrist or finger motion. The utensil can swivel to keep food level.

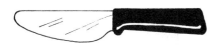

Rocker knife

A *rocker knife* allows for one-handed cutting; several models are available with varying degrees of blade sharpness.

Cups and Glassware

Assisted or independent drinking can be made much safer and easier by using the correct equipment. With impaired oral-motor function, the risk of taking fluid into the lungs can increase. Using a cup that maintains the correct head and neck position during drinking can prevent aspiration. Recall that the recommended position for eating or drinking is with the chin tucked. Here are some options for cups and glasses:

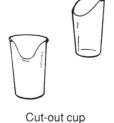

Cut-out cup

Cut-out plastic cups have a piece removed for the person's nose. This allows the person to drink without tipping the head back or extending the neck. These cups are especially helpful for maintaining correct position and monitoring how much liquid is being given.

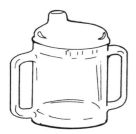

Two-handled mug with lid

Two-handled mugs encourage two-handed drinking.

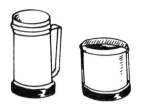

Large-handled mug

Large-handled mugs make holding a mug easier for clients with limited or weak grasp.

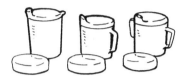

Cups with lids or spouts

Cups with lids or spouts are available in several styles to decrease spillage. Plastic cups generally are much safer for people who have developmental disabilities because these persons tend to have bite reflexes or difficulty with oral movements.

Additional Aids

Non-slip materials of various sorts are available for placing under plates, cups, or glasses to decrease sliding.

For individuals who assist in meal preparation, numerous choices in adaptive cookware can be ordered from catalogs (see resource section). Consult with a therapist to get appropriate suggestions.

Feeding equipment for young children

Positioning during feeding is again a major concern with the younger child. The feeding utensil may need to be smaller as well. Using unbreakable shallow-bowled plastic spoons is recommended.

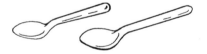

Unbreakable shallow, small-bowled spoons

Feeding Equipment Inventory

The following checklist can be copied for each client to inform all staff of the person's adaptive equipment and positioning needs.

Client's name: _____

Food/liquid consistencies: _____

The following items are to be used during meals in order to promote good eating and drinking skills.

Plates

_____ Plate guard

_____ High-sided plate
type: _____
_____

_____ Scooper bowl

_____ Inner lip plate

Utensils

_____ Built-up handle

_____ Curved handle

_____ Weighted utensils

_____ Swivel utensils

_____ Universal cuff

_____ Rocker knife

Cups/Glassware

_____ Cut-out cup

_____ Two-handled mug

_____ Large-handled mug

_____ Cup with lid

Other

_____ Non-slip material

_____

_____

Positioning Recommendations (To be completed by the consulting therapist)

Copyright © 1991 by Cindy French, Robin Tapp González, and Jan Tronson-Simpson
Published by Therapy Skill Builders, a division of The Psychological Corporation. All rights reserved.
1-800-211-8378 / ISBN 0761647058

8
Dental Hygiene

Since so many of your clients have severe and multifaceted handicaps, they frequently cannot manage their own dental care. The prevention and treatment of dental disorders is vital because neglecting the health of one's mouth can be a source of pain, infection, and odor, which can contribute to feeding difficulties and deter social interaction. Healthy teeth also significantly improve a person's appearance. The way your clients are perceived by others can significantly influence the frequency and type of interaction they receive. However, several factors increase the risk that people with multiple disabilities will develop dental problems:

1. Natural gum stimulators in the diet—such as crunchy foods—would normally help to rid the teeth of bacteria build-up and prevent gum infections. Many individuals with oral-motor involvement, however, cannot tolerate these food textures.

2. Poor tongue and mouth movements may fail to clear food from between the gums and cheeks, as well as allowing particles to become wedged between teeth.

3. Structural abnormalities, such as a high, arched palate or irregularly angled teeth, and poor swallowing skills may make it more difficult to clear food from the mouth.

4. The person may be taking medications regularly to prevent seizures and infections. Some drugs have side effects that damage the tissue (gums) surrounding the teeth. For example, Dilantin®—a drug used to control seizures—can cause extra tissue to grow around the teeth, tissue which must be removed surgically. Careful brushing may help slow the growth of unwanted tissue. Liquid medicines

may damage the teeth because they contain lots of sugar. Liquids containing only 10% sugar can begin cavity formation; yet liquid medications consist, on average, of nearly 50% sugar. Young children with seizures and cerebral palsy may consume almost five pounds of sugar a year from oral liquid medication alone! No wonder health care professionals prescribe medications in tablet form as soon as possible!

5. Because of seizures or poor motor coordination, clients may fall and damage their teeth or the tissue in their mouths.

You should know about two common disease processes: tooth decay and gum disease, also known as *periodontal disease* or *pyorrhea.* Both problems are usually caused by a build-up of *plaque.* Plaque is a gummy film infested with bacteria. These bacteria produce acids that dissolve the *enamel,* the outside surface of the teeth, and also destroy the surface of the gums, causing bleeding. If plaque is not removed daily, the bacteria spread deeper and destroy the bone that supports the teeth. If this happens, the only treatment is pulling teeth.

There are two ways to control tooth decay and bleeding gums:

1. Cut down on the amount of sugar the person eats. The bacteria in plaque change the sugar to acid in order to attack the teeth and gums.

2. Brush the teeth and gums thoroughly every day.

Environmental Considerations

The first thing to think about when planning good dental care is the surroundings. Personal care should take place in a natural environment. This means that you need to consider these factors:

1. Each person, regardless of disability, should be given privacy.

2. Rid the area of unnecessary distractions.

3. Allow the individual as much independence as possible. In most cases, you will have to brush the teeth to be sure they are properly cleaned, but don't miss opportunities for the client to participate. If possible, allow the person to choose the color of the toothbrush or cup to be used. If possible, help the individual hold the toothbrush, put it in the mouth, and brush.

4. Whether you are supervising or carrying out the task, explain what you are doing.

Positioning Considerations

1. Keep the individual as upright as possible. If the person must recline, it's better to recline the upper trunk rather than hyperextending the neck.

2. Use the same position you would for feeding, if possible.

3. Remember, by introducing a stimulant (the toothbrush) into the mouth, you will be increasing salivation and the need for swallowing. Yet, having a toothbrush in the mouth can make it difficult to coordinate swallowing with breathing, which puts the person at risk for choking. Moreover, tipping the head back can create a choking feeling and cause the person to panic.

4. For individuals who are hypersensitive to touch (see chapters 5 and 7), tooth brushing can be very difficult to tolerate. Giving external oral stimulation (see chapter 7) just prior to tooth brushing may help in completing the task.

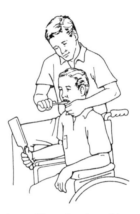 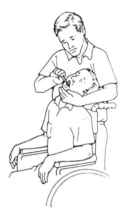

Correct position for brushing teeth. Placing a mirror in front of the client will allow you to see into the person's mouth without tipping the head back.

Incorrect position for brushing teeth. Tipping the head back may cause the person to choke.

Equipment

A soft-bristled toothbrush is recommended. The water should be at room temperature. As discussed in chapter 5, either hot or cold temperatures can be difficult for your clients to tolerate. Toothpaste is *not* recommended. This comes as a surprise to many care providers and parents. Toothpaste causes suds and increased salivation in the mouth, which can contribute to swallowing problems. The cleansing action actually comes from the brushing itself, not from the use of toothpaste. Moreover, swallowing toothpaste causes constipation. Toothpaste serves only as a breath freshener. After you have carefully brushed the teeth, you can place a small amount of toothpaste on the tongue in order to freshen breath. An alternative is to occasionally dip the toothbrush in a liquid dentifrice (tooth cleaner)—several are on the market. If possible let the individual choose the flavor of the tooth cleaner. A person with adequate motor and visual skills could participate by holding a hand mirror.

Brushing Techniques

Technique is important. Clients can pick up from your handling and approach whether you are confident about completing the task and how you regard them as individuals. Try to use a gentle, yet firm and respectful approach. Having their teeth brushed is not a favorite activity for many clients, yet it is a very important hygiene task.

Suggestions

It usually works best to brush all the upper teeth, and then move to the lower teeth (or vice versa), rather than brushing the top teeth on one side, then moving to the bottom teeth, then returning to the top, and so on. The brush should be placed so that the head of the brush rests against the lips with the bristles pointing toward the gums.

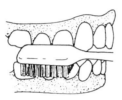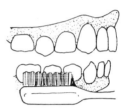

Brush placement for tooth brushing

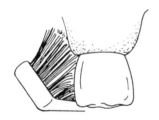

Notice the 45-degree angle between the toothbrush bristles and the teeth, with the bristles touching the teeth and gums.

Then turn the brush inward, which rolls the bristles into contact with the teeth. There should be about a 45-degree angle between the bristles and the teeth, and the bristles should be touching the gums.

This way, the tooth surface and gums are brushed at the same time. The brush should be moved up and down six to eight strokes for each tooth. Clean the cheek side of the teeth, then complete the same procedure on the tongue side of the same arch. If necessary, remove the toothbrush and allow the person a chance to swallow, then repeat the entire process on the opposing arch.

Although most of us have been taught that we should brush our teeth following each meal or snack, some dental experts advocate brushing before the meal or before giving liquid medication. In this way, the bacteria are removed from the teeth before the meal. Whichever procedure you follow, the most important factor is that the teeth are consistently, routinely, and thoroughly brushed at least two times daily. If the client eats sweets, you should brush more often.

This chapter has given you the basic information you need to take good care of your clients' teeth and gums. Remember that routine dental checkups are very important, especially for people who cannot take care of their own teeth and may not be able to tell you that they have a toothache. Please refer to your dental professional for additional information to supplement the guidelines in this chapter.

9
Bathing and Dressing

Two areas of self-care that people with normal motor skills take for granted are bathing and dressing. These self-care tasks are automatic to most of us. A person with severe disabilities will require assistance with these tasks, however, or may even require total care. Regardless of the level of participation each person is capable of, as a caregiver you can provide therapeutic handling and some opportunities for clients to assist themselves.

Bathing

As you prepare an area for a bath, consider these factors:

1. How comfortable is the water temperature? Warm water relaxes muscles, which is especially helpful for an individual with high tone.

2. Are supplies within easy reach? It is important not to disrupt a bath in the middle to fetch additional supplies, especially as doing so could put you and the client at risk for injury.

3. Is the room warm? The beneficial effects of a warm bath will be lost quickly if the person becomes chilled after getting out of the tub.

4. If bathtub positioning equipment is used, is it in working order, and does it have safety restraints? Just as with any positioning equipment, a good safety belt is warranted and should always be used.

5. If the client draws the bath water, are safeguards in place to prevent the water being too hot? There are several ways to reduce risk—for example, turning down a hot water heater or purchasing commercial products that regulate water temperature.

6. Are towels and equipment ready for assisting the individual out of the bath or shower? This transition should be completed as smoothly and quickly as possible. Large beach towels provide more drying area, and they can be placed on the floor, a changing surface, or an adaptive chair. Then the client can be assisted to the towel, wrapped in it, and dried.

As you help a client to undress before a bath, you can take the opportunity to incorporate some therapeutic movement activities. You can relax the muscles of clients with high tone by rotating the upper part of the body on the lower part. Rotation also is useful in taking off pants or slacks:

1. Bend the persons's hips and knees toward the chest.

2. Turn the legs to one side as you pull the pants off one hip.

3. Turn the legs to the opposite side, then pull the pants down over that hip.

4. Bring the pants down the person's legs with the legs rotated to one side, if possible. Rotate the legs to the opposite side as needed.

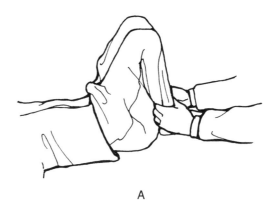

A

Bend the person's hips and knees toward the chest.

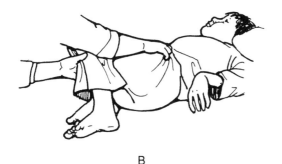

B

Turn the legs to one side as you pull the pants off the top hip.

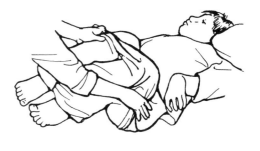

C

Then rotate the legs to the other side and pull the pants off the other hip.

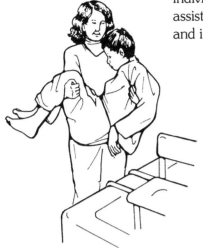

Transferring, or moving the individual into and out of the bath can be easy or difficult. One caretaker can safely assist a small or lightweight individual; two people may be needed for larger clients. If the individual assists with transfers, you should be familiar with how to promote safety and independence. Below are some examples of bathroom transfers:

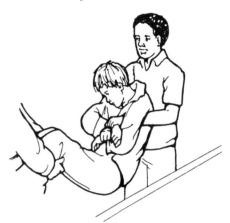

One-person carry to transfer a small person into a bathtub

Two-person transfer

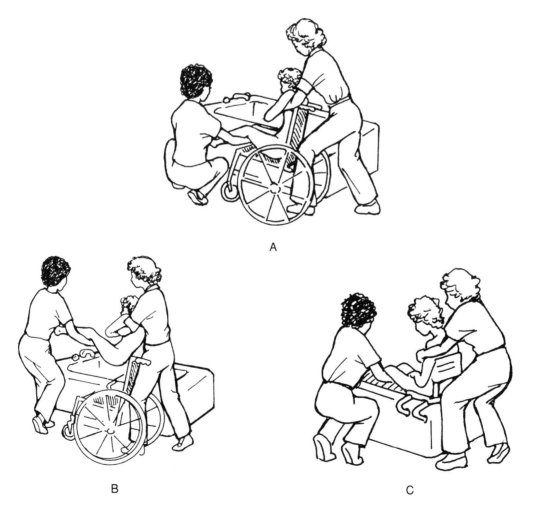

A

B

C

Two-person transfer from a wheelchair to a tub bench

Adaptive Equipment

Several adaptive equipment options are available. Grab bars of several types can be installed inside the tub or shower stall. A bath chair is a good choice for the client who needs sitting support. If a client requires only partial assistance and sits with good balance, a tub bench or a rolling shower chair may be recommended.

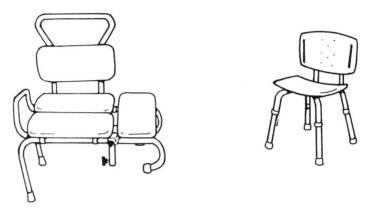

Examples of shower and tub chairs

Promoting client participation should be your primary concern. Using a bath mitt may encourage an individual with limited motor movements to try to wash. If reaching is a problem, a long-handled sponge may be used. Water play is fun for people of all ages. For younger clients, a variety of toys can encourage motor movements and teach cause-and-effect relationships. Just remember how much fun it was to "sink" the rubber ducky! Bath time can also be a time to let the client make choices and to stimulate language. It's great to encourage singing in the shower.

Dressing

Assisting an individual with severe disabilities to dress and undress can be a definite challenge. Clothing selection, positioning, client participation, and handling techniques all must be considered. These areas will be discussed and general guidelines provided.

Clothing selection

The choice of clothing may appear unimportant until you are asked to assist a client in putting on a pullover shirt that is too small in the neck and the sleeves. Here are some guidelines to keep in mind:

1. Clothes that open down the front are generally easier to put on and take off.

2. Look for fuller clothing styles, ones with larger neck openings and dolman or raglan sleeves.

3. Choose fabrics that "give" or stretch slightly.

4. Avoid fabrics that feel itchy or rough.

5. Short jackets, capes, or ponchos are easier for clients in wheelchairs.

6. Breathable fabrics, such as cotton and other natural fibers, are more comfortable.

Positioning

Try to position clients so they can assist you with dressing. It's important for clients to feel that they have a role in their self-care, rather than feeling that every activity is being done to them. Talk with the occupational and physical therapists to get additional ideas of how individual clients can participate. Here are some examples:

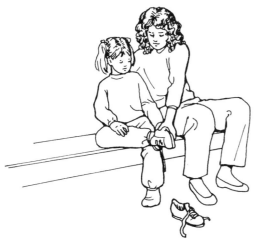

Putting on a girl's shoes in supported sitting on a bench. Crossing the legs keeps the toes from curling and makes it easier to put the shoe on.

- Rolling from back lying to sidelying on a bed or mat promotes muscle tone relaxation and purposeful movement. Help a client roll from side to side while you (or the client) pull up slacks, tights, or a diaper. Refer back to page 86 to refresh your memory on the technique.
- Putting on or taking off shoes and socks may be easiest in supported sitting on an adapted seat.
- Supported sitting on a bench may be an appropriate dressing position for a client with good balance.

Client participation

All clients can be encouraged to assist with dressing or undressing, whether they provide little assistance or are mostly independent. Depending on individual capabilities, here are ways of involving clients:

- Let them make choices such as color or style of clothing.
- Ask them to sequence the task, to indicate or tell you what goes on first, then second, and so on.
- Encourage them to move in more normal patterns, for example, straightening an arm that is usually bent.
- Ask them to complete part of a task, for example, pulling up a sock after you maneuver it past the heel.

As you assist a client with dressing, here are some general guidelines based on therapy techniques:

1. When pulling clothing over a client's head, position the head with the neck flexed and some chin tuck, rather than letting the neck go into extension.

2. Try to keep the person's head in midline.

3. If one side of the body has more muscle tone (is stiffer), put the more spastic arm or leg into clothing first. As a general rule, dress the limb with less mobility before the limb with greater movement.

4. The more involved arm or leg should be taken out of clothing after the better limb.

5. Do not "pull" on a tight arm to help the person get into a coat or shirt; insert the arm into the sleeve as far as you can, then run your hand into the sleeve and help the individual straighten the arm, while you help pull up the sleeve.

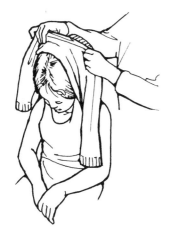

Try to keep the head and neck bent forward when taking off or putting on shirts.

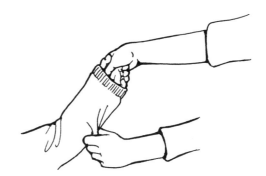

Give assistance by helping the person to straighten his or her arm while you push the sleeve down.

6. If an individual's muscles are tight, remember that good positioning can help. If a client's toes curl as you try to put on shoes, bend the hip and knee and cross one leg over the other, if possible. This position relaxes high muscle tone and may help with putting shoes on.

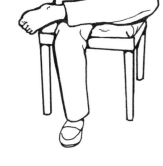

Bending the hip and knee and, if possible, crossing the leg can help relax tight muscles. This will help you put on socks or shoes.

Your clients will need assistance with areas of self-care you probably take for granted. Things like choosing clothing, making sure you have all bathing supplies in advance, and positioning and transferring the client correctly may seem to be unimportant details. However, they will make personal care more efficient for you and more pleasant for the client, will allow the client to perform more tasks independently, and may prevent injury to you or the client.

10

Communication

Communication refers to the act of sharing information. It's a means of expressing ideas, information, feelings, and desires through which we teach and learn new skills. Not communicating is impossible, because any behavior transmits information, whether or not we wish it to do so. Facial expression, posture, and choice of clothing all communicate messages about us without our saying even one word.

Speech and *language* are subcategories of communication. An explanation of terms will help you understand the specific abilities needed to develop speech and language. *Speech* refers to the production of sounds using the mouth, the quality of voice, and the rhythm of the words. The abilities needed to develop speech are visibly functioning at birth. The coordinated mouth and face movements a newborn uses for nursing, breathing, and crying are the building blocks for producing voice and forming individual sounds; later these sounds will be put together to make words and sentences. All the parts of the body that are used in speaking have primary purposes other than speech (namely to meet survival needs such as breathing and eating), so the infant immediately begins "practicing" skills that will be used for speech. These skills include swallowing; sucking; moving the lips, jaw, and tongue; and regulating and coordinating breathing.

Speech is one of the most complex functions the body performs because so many muscles are involved—more than 100! It shouldn't be surprising, then, that a person who has difficulty with large body movements often also has difficulty with the small, detailed movements needed for speech. A person who can make only limited mouth movements won't be able to make all the sounds we use in English (called the *sound inventory* of English). The sounds the person can make will be those that require little or no tongue or lip movements, and many sounds will be distorted. The person is more likely to make vowel sounds than consonant sounds. Say "ah," and compare it to "sss." Note the difference in the mouth movements needed.

Three abilities are needed for speech development:

1. Good motor (movement) control and coordination of the mouth, throat, and breathing muscles

2. The ability to hear and distinguish the differences among sounds

3. Adequate thinking skills to put the sounds together accurately and meaningfully

Individual speech sounds are put together into a symbol system, called *language* that is used to express thoughts and feelings. A *symbol* is something that a group of people agree stands for something else, as speakers of English agree that the word "car" stands for a vehicle used for transportation. Language symbols can be verbal, gestural, written, or pictorial. For example, if someone says "eat," we know that this combination of sounds ($\bar{e}$ + t) means the process of taking in food. However, a person could also gesture "eat," or point to a picture of someone eating to convey the same meaning.

Children learn language from their everyday interactions with objects, toys, parents and peers, movement, and experiences with the different senses. Verbal language is the fastest and most efficient way to communicate; there are, as you saw in the previous example, alternatives to verbal language, such as signing or pointing to pictures or written words. Simply because an individual has limited physical abilities to speak, don't assume that they cannot understand what you say or use language in some other, unspoken, form.

Language can be further divided into two areas, *receptive language* and *expressive language.* Receptive language refers to the ability to understand a message. It can be as basic as stopping an activity in response to sound or as complex as studying for a physics exam. A baby first learns to locate where a sound is coming from (called *localization*). Then the baby learns to pay attention to certain sounds—for example, babies prefer to listen to someone talking than to other environmental sounds. Gradually the baby begins associating objects, actions, and feelings with words. This is a beginning skill for understanding the meaning of words. A baby gains all these receptive language skills before saying even one word.

Expressive language refers to the ability to convey a message, through either speech, gestures, or an *augmentative/alternative communication system,* such as signing, pointing to pictures on a communication board, or using a computer system with voice output. Expressive language can be as basic as smiling when you are happy or as complex as speaking in a foreign language. It includes interaction skills as well—responding when someone interacts with you, initiating interaction with someone, keeping an interaction going, and taking turns in a conversation.

Prelanguage skills are skills a baby or child learns before using the first "real," meaningful word, whether spoken or nonverbal. Many of our clients, who are multiply handicapped and severely to profoundly involved, function in the prespeech and prelanguage stage of development. As with speech, one's ability to use language is greatly influenced by the level of one's thinking skills. Although not all of our clients have the ability to master a symbol system, they can learn to communicate more usefully with you. Better communication will enrich their lives by allowing them to contribute to their environment and have some form of control over what is going on around them. That is exactly the goal of communication—to have a way of controlling our environment so that we can shape our surroundings to best suit us. Imagine how helpless you would feel if you were cold and hungry but didn't have a way to ask anyone for a blanket and food.

You will learn to communicate and interact only if people in the environment respond to you. Because of their severe physical and mental disabilities, your clients may not seem to respond to or communicate with you. It's easy to get frustrated and give up when your clients make such slow progress. In turn, when you get discouraged, you talk with and communicate with your clients less often, which gives them fewer opportunities to communicate with you, even though they need just the opposite.

Tips for Increasing Communication throughout the Day

1. Be a good observer. Notice small, subtle body or facial movements individuals may use when they are uncomfortable, when they like something, or when they don't like something. Remember, your clients can communicate with you without meaning to. Notice which types of stimulation the person responds to best and most consistently—for example, sounds, touch, or sights.

2. Notice consistent responses. For example, say you notice that every time you try to feed a client cooked carrots, the individual turns away from the spoon and tightly closes her or his mouth. Chances are pretty good that the person doesn't like carrots. You will want to respond by giving meaning to the behavior—"You don't like cooked carrots." Keep track of all likes and dislikes you notice so you can have a better understanding of the person and can offer appropriate choices.

3. Arrange each day's activities in a predictable routine. This helps the individual learn that there is a beginning and an ending to each daily activity. After learning the routine, the person may start to participate in it, and perhaps even initiate the next step. Suppose that following each meal, you wash the client's hands and face and wipe the lap tray. Is the individual able to wipe the tray, or at least help with the task?

4. Frequently give the client names for objects, activities, and feelings. Even a client who never uses these words may learn to understand them and respond to them.

5. Whenever possible, offer your clients choices. Make sure that you offer choices only when either choice is acceptable and possible for the client. Then go ahead and follow through with the chosen item or activity. Even a very involved person can make a slight body or eye movement to communicate a choice. Here are some choices you might offer:

   - A choice between two clothing items (a red shirt or a green shirt)
   - A choice of dishes or cups at mealtime
   - A choice of musical instruments during a group activity
   - A choice between two after-shave fragrances for males or two hair combs for females.

6. Focus on things that the person wants and needs to communicate. For instance, signaling the desire for "toilet" may be very useful for you, but it has little value for the person. The person probably has much more interest in signaling the desire for a cookie (or a favorite game). When you're trying to teach a person to communicate, look for signs or words that give some immediate power over the environment and are motivating enough to be reinforcing: If I sign "toilet," what do I get? But if I sign "cookie," I get a yummy treat. Once the person has begun to communicate, you can begin to teach less concrete and rewarding ideas like "toilet." If the person uses undesirable or unacceptable behavior as a means of signaling something, offer an alternative means of communicating the same feeling.

7. The physical and manipulative skills you teach clients when you help them feed and care for themselves are skills they might be able to use later to access a communication device.

8. Be aware of the individual's body position. Remember that an abnormal body position may give you fewer language experiences. If you were always lying down, or if your head were drooping on your chest or tipped sideways out of a wheelchair, you wouldn't be able to watch the activities and people around you, or you wouldn't be able to see them in the way most people do. Thus, a person who has a severe disability may not be able to observe the connection between a sound and its source, and the same principle is true for

the other senses of sight, smell, and touch. Just positioning clients properly can greatly enhance the stimulation that is around them, as well as helping them interpret its meaning.

Communication is a way of sharing information. It is also a very redundant process, which can help (or confuse) a person in understanding a given message. We choose appropriate words, facial expressions, body gestures and mannerisms, and perhaps even clothing to help get our messages across. For instance, imagine a lawyer in a courtroom defending a client—not only does she carefully choose her words, but her facial expression tells us she is serious. The way she stands, her posture and pacing style, and the clothing she chooses all give us information. Now imagine the lawyer giving exactly the same speech, but grinning widely throughout it, or walking with an exaggerated sway in her hips, or being dressed in an evening gown. Do you think she would convey the same message, even though she used exactly the same words?

The point of this example is that for someone who is developmentally delayed, many of the redundancies of communication are changed or absent. Frequently, the person cannot use speech, or the usual rhythm of speech and pronunciation of words may be changed due to difficulty with breathing or coordinating the muscles in the mouth. Due to changes in muscle tone and the way different movements and positions affect other parts of the body, facial expressions may be absent or may not match the intent of the message. Touching someone who has tactile defensiveness may cause a startle that results in unintentional body movements or facial expressions.

General Language Stimulation

Language stimulation is one way of providing active treatment. As you will recall, *active treatment* is a method of promoting interaction and teaching the client to be an active participant in the environment. Language stimulation is easier than it sounds, because language is everywhere. Even when you don't think you're teaching language, you are, because language includes laughter, words, gestures, signs, body movements, facial expressions, and tones of voice. Here are some ways you can stimulate language:

1. Be aware of how you provide for the basic needs of the person you are caring for. Your attitude, expression, voice, words, and handling methods are the first bridge for building trust and warmth in a relationship.

2. Give the person a rich background of words and experiences to draw from. Use exciting vocabulary. Don't just name and label things, but also talk about characteristics (big, pretty), actions (wash, eat), and feelings. Give the person an opportunity to experience these things in the environment as often as possible, using all the senses.

Encourage watching, touching, hearing, feeling, smelling, and tasting things whenever you can.

For example, in dressing you might say, "Which sweater would you like to wear today? Look, (name), here is your smooth black sweater or your fuzzy white sweater." Actually rub each sweater against the person's hand or face and repeat the words "smooth" and "fuzzy." This way the person gets a wide range of sensory experiences in just the activities you do every day.

Another example is to actually make orange juice, rather than simply pouring it from the carton. Show the person the whole orange. Let the client feel its roundness, coldness, and the consistency of the peel. Next, peel or slice it open. Let the individual smell the orange and feel the inside and taste it. Provide words for the characteristics being experienced. Help the person physically interact using a variety of senses.

3. It's best to be at the person's *eye level* when interacting.

4. Provide lots of repetition. Normally developing children require lots of repetition to learn a concept, and so do your clients. Repetition is not boring to them, but rather helps them learn.

5. If the individual has a hearing impairment, keep the object you are talking about near your mouth, so the person can attend to your lips as you talk about it.

6. Have an individual who is visually impaired actually hold an object (with your assistance, if necessary) while you describe it. When a client has a sensory deficit, try to present information through other senses.

Alternative and Augmentative Communication

Alternative communication and augmentative communication are terms that refer to types of communication aids. These terms are frequently used interchangeably, since they both refer to assisting or adapting communication. *Augmentative communication* refers to any method that assists a person to communicate. An augmentative system may be used to supplement a person's limited speech skills in order to clarify or expand the message. *Alternative communication* refers to any means of communicating other than speech. Augmentative communication systems may be simple or complex—gesturing or pointing, sign language, communication boards or books, electronic devices, and computers are examples.

An augmentative or alternative communication system cannot be issued indiscriminately, the way you buy one pair of socks that fits all sizes. Rather, the system is individualized for the specific capabilities and needs of the user. The first step is to refer the individual to trained specialists (usually a speech-language pathologist and an occupational therapist) who can determine whether the individual can benefit from an alternative system and what type of system is most suitable. The evaluation procedure assesses the individual's physical capabilities, motor skills, perceptual skills, language development, thinking skills, educational or vocational needs, and recreational abilities and needs. Once a system has been chosen, several factors relating to maintenance and use have to be considered:

1. Who trains the user *and* everyone who regularly interacts with the user in how to operate the system (whether this involves learning and interpreting sign language or using an electronic device)? If the system requires maintenance, can the user care for it, or do others need to be trained?

2. Is the system accessible in all the user's environments? For instance, if the system is a communication board, is it always available to the user, or is it stuck up on a shelf out of reach?

3. Can the system easily be altered as the individual's needs change? Will it accommodate growth and progress in communication skills (for example, increased vocabulary)?

Once a system has been provided, the user has to learn how to use it as efficiently as possible. You have to have a good working knowledge of the system so you can help your client use it. Frequent and consistent use are the best ways of teaching the user to use the system. Also remember to respond to all attempts to communicate using the system, even if you have to say something like, "I know you want a cookie, but you can't have one right now."

You may also need to learn how to be a "good listener" to the device: How long should you wait for an answer? How should you sit or stand to make the communication as natural as possible? Here are some strategies that will help you:

1. Pay attention to your own nonverbal communication. Does your nonverbal message match your words?

2. Ask short, simple questions, one at a time. Phrase your questions so that responses other than "yes" or "no" can be given. Compare "What do you want to drink?" with "Do you want some juice?"

3. Allow time for a response.

4. Be patient.

5. Know how the person's signaling system or communication device works. Make sure the system is available.

6. Speak in a regular conversational tone, rather than talking down to the person or talking louder than normal. The tone of your voice conveys a lot.

7. Be at eye level whenever possible.

8. Tell the person if you do not understand the message. Do not be afraid to ask the person to repeat the message or give you more information. Making this extra effort to understand a message lets the person know that his or her message is important to you.

9. Respond positively and acknowledge the individual's communicative attempts—this can be as basic as a smile or a touch on the arm.

Summary

Many things have to be considered in establishing a successful communicative environment, regardless of how the person communicates. Communication is an interactive process that has to be a part of your client's daily life. Positioning, providing movement and support, and attending to verbal and nonverbal cues are very important factors that you cannot overlook. No matter what you are doing, you can encourage the client to communicate with you.

If your client communicates with sounds, remember to allow for a good breathing pattern. The airway needs to be straight between the rib cage and the mouth, and the client has to be in a stable posture. If the individual has to point to, look at, touch, or attend to some kind of communicative device, place the device so the user can see and reach it easily given his or her physical limitations. Notice how well the person you work with is able to respond to you in different positions. (See chapter 11 on switch mechanisms for more information.)

Although the person you are working with probably does not produce words or many sounds, communication is no less important. Body movement, facial expression, eye contact, and other responses can be first attempts at communication. Be a good observer and watch for different responses. Always try to be sensitive to the individual's feelings and experiences in a situation. Your voice is an important tool that you always carry with you. Remember to talk about what you are doing in a pleasant conversational tone as you move and position the person. Whenever possible, speak face-to-face. This may mean sitting down at eye level with the person. Communicate whenever you can, both verbally and nonverbally. Use facial expression and touch—every possible way to communicate.

11
Switch Mechanisms

A *switch* is an access device used to gain some form of control over the environment. Adaptive switches can be powered by a wind-up mechanism, by batteries, or by electrical current. You may not even realize the wide variety of switches we use routinely—such as an ordinary light switch. The light switch is one example of how we can adapt an energy source. The light switch provides access to electrical current and harnesses it in a useful manner. Operating an electric toothbrush, running the garbage disposer, turning on a fan, or operating a remote-control race car are all examples of how we can use switches to control our surroundings for work and recreational activities.

Individuals with limited mobility usually have had little opportunity or experience in controlling anything in their environments. Following a complete evaluation of these individuals' environments, their communication skills and needs, and body movement options, however, a switch or other adaptive device may be found that allows them to control some part of their world. This control could be as simple as using a switch to operate a toy or as complex as accessing a computer.

Purpose of Switch Use

1. A switch enables a person to be more independent by controlling some part of the environment. This control can lead to better self-help, educational, communication, and leisure skills. For example, a person could use switches to move an electrical feeder, operate a blender to mix a milk shake, turn on a tape recording, or communicate using a voice produced by a computer.

2. For a person who is nonverbal, the purpose of a switch may be as basic as signaling for attention or responding *yes* or *no*. Or, a switch can control a high-tech communication system that allows the person to hold conversations.

3. Using a switch can encourage purposeful movement and better movement skills. For example, the user may learn to keep the head upright and in midline or to reach across midline with one hand. (This movement is very difficult for many people with severe physical disabilities.)

4. A switch can be used for teaching cause-and-effect relationships, which is a basic thinking skill.

5. Switches can help to teach things we take for granted: how to use and play with objects and how to pay attention, as well as all sorts of sensory experiences.

6. Many of your clients may *self-stimulate* in ways that can hurt them, such as head banging. Switches can cut down on this kind of behavior by letting individuals focus on a purposeful action they can control and repeat.

Types of Switches

Switches come in many different shapes, sizes, and types and can be operated in a wide variety of ways. (No matter how the switch works, its purpose remains the same—to access and control a device.) Because so many different types of switches are available, only the basic types will be outlined here. Many different ready-made switches are available, and almost any type of switch can be made at home with parts bought at an electronics store. Several instructional books on the market explain how to make switches and adapt toys, appliances, and educational devices for switch use, as well as providing ideas for using switches.

Push switches

Push switches are probably the most widely used. They come in several different styles, but they are all *activated* (turned on and off) using some degree of pressure. They may be resistant or extremely sensitive to touch. Most switches make a clicking sound when they are activated to provide additional feedback to the user. Continuous pressure is needed to keep the device operating. A push switch can be mounted so that any part of the body can operate it. The examples on the following page show the wide variety of switches that are available.

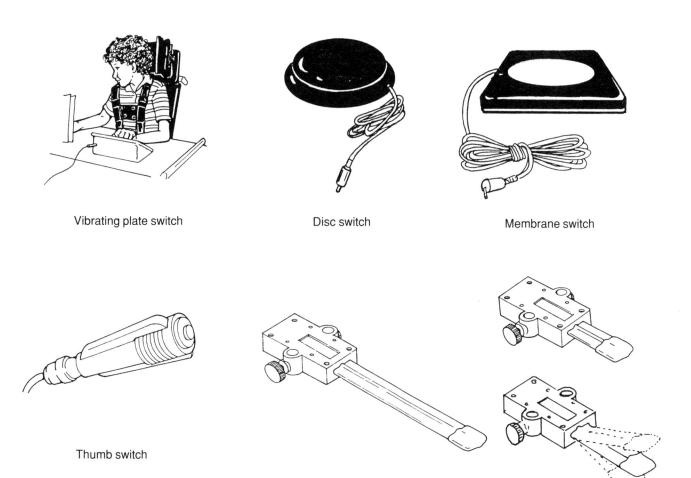

Vibrating plate switch

Disc switch

Membrane switch

Thumb switch

Lever switches

Pneumatic switches

A pneumatic switch is operated by increasing or decreasing air pressure. Two common types of pneumatic switches are the *sip-and-puff* switch and the *squeeze-ball* switch—activated by squeezing a ball or puffing to increase pressure or sipping to decrease it.

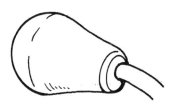

Pneumatic switch

Mercury switches

A mercury switch is activated when movement causes the mercury inside a casing to make contact with a metal prong. This switch is fastened to some part of the body (usually the head) and is activated with movement. Mercury switches are typically attached to headbands, barrettes, or hats.

Joysticks

A joystick is activated through directional movement. Joysticks are often used to control the movement of electric wheelchairs.

Push-on/push-off switches

A push-on/push-off switch is similar to the push switches described previously, except that one push turns the device on, and it remains on until the switch is pushed a second time to turn it off. Continuous pressure is not needed to keep the device on.

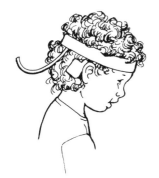

Mercury switch on a headband

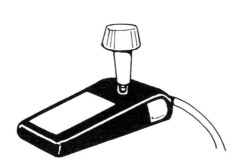

Joystick

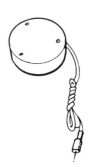

Push on/push off switch

Voice-activated switches

A voice-activated switch is activated in response to the client's voice.

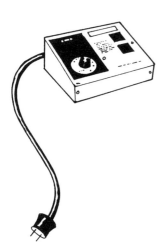

Control unit

Another adaptive device that is helpful and can be used with any type of switch is a *control unit*. A control unit acts as an interface to allow electrical appliances to be accessed by a switch. It may be equipped with a timer for someone who has difficulty maintaining pressure on the switch; each time the switch is tripped, the attached device will stay activated for a preset length of time. A timer is useful for activating objects like radios and tape recorders, which may be damaged or give a distorted signal if rapidly and repeatedly turned on and off.

Positioning

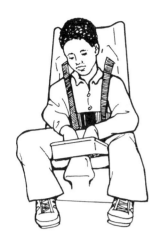

A client using an augmentative system in adaptive seating.

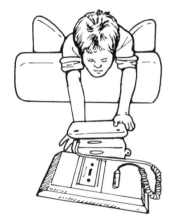

A client using a switch to activate a tape recorder while positioned on his stomach on a wedge.

As with any activity requiring voluntary movement, positioning of the user is important (see chapter 6). A switch can be activated from a variety of positions. Sidelying with good support, stomach lying on a wedge, or sitting in a corner chair or bolster chair may all be suitable alternatives to sitting in a wheelchair. The therapist(s) involved with your client will be glad to assist you in identifying effective positions. Here are some factors to consider when positioning an individual:

1. What position will facilitate the motion needed to activate the switch?

2. Does the position inhibit abnormal reflexes?
   - Is the client's head in midline?
   - Is the head in a neutral or slightly flexed position?

3. Does the position also promote other goals, such as better head control?

4. Does the user have a good visual field while looking straight ahead or slightly down?

5. Encourage an appropriate movement. Is the motion needed to activate the switch useful for other tasks as well? Will it cause other undesirable reactions in the body?

6. Position the user and the switch so that the person can see, feel, hear, or touch the object being activated.

7. Use an object that is appropriate to the age and capability of the person. Choose an object that motivates the client to respond.

Summary

In conclusion, switches are one kind of adaptive device that can be used to modify or to bypass conventional methods of using electronic devices. They provide alternative ways for people with disabilities to interact with their surroundings and gain some control over their environment. Using a switch can increase sensory input, provide environmental control, aid in developing recreation and leisure skills, develop cognitive, motor, and communication skills, and provide an acceptable method of self-stimulation. Switch training may be an end in itself or it may be a stage in learning to operate computerized communication systems and other functional devices, such as an electric wheelchair. An individual's environmental needs, communication needs and skills, and body movements are all evaluated to determine the most suitable device.

12
Fine Motor Guidelines

Fine motor skills begin with a child learning to use the hands and arms to reach and grasp objects, on which basis are built more complex and precise skills. As you will recall from the introduction, *fine motor* refers to skilled movements that require use of the small muscles of the hands, arms, and mouth. Fine motor skills are influenced by many things—vision, muscle tone, strength, coordination, and general posture. Take, for example, cutting a circle from a piece of paper with scissors and think of all the steps you must be able to complete:

- Pick up the scissors and correctly place your fingers in the handles.
- Pick up the paper and turn it to the place where you want to start cutting.
- Coordinate opening and closing the scissors with turning the paper at the right moment to stay on the outline of the circle.

This simple task involves vision, grasping both the scissors and paper in appropriate ways, coordinating the muscles of the hands and arms, eye/hand coordination, and timing, all while sitting in a chair without falling over. We often take a "simple" skill like this for granted. For an individual with a motor handicap, this "easy" activity can range from frustrating to nearly impossible.

Therapists or teachers, particularly occupational therapists, often evaluate the fine motor skills of clients with physical handicaps. From such an assessment, they make recommendations to improve problem areas or help the individual adapt tasks to compensate for fine motor difficulties. Their goals might cover a variety of areas, including the following:

- To improve trunk control
- To increase muscle tone in a client with low muscle tone
- To assist the individual with high muscle tone to move more easily
- To hold large joints (such as the shoulder) steady
- To develop mature grasp and release of objects
- To develop better coordination between vision and hand movements
- To use both hands together
- To improve general coordination and strength

Here are some general guidelines to follow when setting up a fine motor activity and assisting clients to complete it:

1. Position the client in a chair or piece of adaptive equipment that gives good support. Imagine being asked to pour liquid into a glass while your body was tipped to one side. Having your trunk off balance would make pouring much more difficult. This is the experience of clients who have poor trunk or head and neck control.

2. Similarly, if the muscle tone is different on the two sides of a person's body—for example, if the muscles are tighter on one side of the body—this difference can make fine motor tasks difficult. Assist a client with an imbalance (sometimes called an *asymmetry*) by making sure the legs are supported evenly; the hips are even; the trunk is supported; and both arms are forward, preferably supported on a tray or tabletop.

3. Be aware that the person's sight may not be good. Choose objects that contrast sharply—for example, place a dark object against a light background—to help the person see the object more clearly. Or use objects that make sound.

4. Remind clients to look at objects before reaching for them, and help them keep their attention on the task at hand.

5. Try to present objects so your clients can reach for them with the thumb and palm up. This type of reach is a more mature grasping pattern.

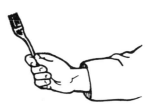

Thumb and palm-up grasp

6. Encourage grasp on the thumb side of the hand (called the *radial side*), rather than on the little-finger side.

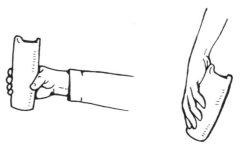

Illustrations of thumb side (radial) grasp (left)
and little-finger side (ulnar) grasp (right)

7. Talk to the occupational therapist about the best size of object to use. Different sizes and shapes require use of different grasping patterns.

As you notice difficulties a client has, the therapy team can show you activities that will help the client progress. Some of the activities may help the individual to experience how it feels to move in a more normal way. Or you may be teaching the person to use special equipment such as modified scissors. Or you may be encouraging the person to grasp an object in a better way. It is important for primary caretakers to know, not only *how* to complete the exercise or activity, but also *why* they are doing it. It is just as important to respect clients' right to know the purpose of activities that are done with them. Explain the activity to the individual in whatever way you can to encourage cooperation. Giving the client and the therapist feedback about progress is always helpful.

Splinting

A splint (also called an *orthotic*) is a plastic or metal support that is specially made for an individual to help protect, support, or correct the position of a body part or to assist with a specific function, such as holding a pencil. A splint is generally made by an occupational or physical therapist or an orthotist and is custom molded for the client from a heat-sensitive plastic. Therefore, you should *never* switch splints among clients or try a splint on a person other than the one for whom it was made.

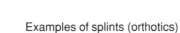

Examples of splints (orthotics)

There are two types of splints, static and dynamic; either type is strapped onto the client. *Static splints* have no movable parts and generally help position, support, or protect an area. *Dynamic splints* have movable parts, and may require setup and adjustment by a therapist. If a client uses a splint, you should ask the prescribing therapist for the following information:

- Why is the splint being made?
- Which arm or leg is the splint for? If the client uses two hand splints, clearly mark the splints "left" and "right."
- When should the client wear the splint? It's a good idea to write out a schedule. Does the client need to wear the splint for short periods at first to accept and tolerate it?
- How do I clean or care for the splint?
- How do I put on and remove the splint? Ask for a photo or drawing that shows the correct way to put on the splint. Also make sure that more than one person knows how to put the splint on properly.
- Are there other exercises I should do while the client is wearing the splint?

Here are some problems you should be on the lookout for. If you notice a problem, immediately take off the splint and notify the therapist before using it again:

- Redness or chafing of the skin underneath the splint or straps
- Pain or discomfort
- Stiffness
- Pressure areas or sores, especially under the splint
- Swelling
- Major difficulty putting on the orthotic

Keep splints away from heat sources because heat will make them change shape. Don't leave a splint in a hot car or next to a stove, radiator, or other heat source, and don't try to wash it in a washing machine or dishwasher, or even in hot water.

If the orthotic is to be worn most of the day, it should be removed at intervals to do range of motion exercises on the limb, unless the therapist tells you differently.

If you have *any* questions about how to put on a splint or how long the individual is to wear it, please contact the therapist. It is always better to leave a splint off for a few hours than to accidentally cause an individual discomfort by using the device incorrectly.

13
Gross Motor Guidelines

Gross motor development is the process of learning to move from one place to another. It is a process regulated by the maturing brain, and it occurs in a beautiful, well-planned sequence. Normal children progress smoothly from one stage of motor development to another. Babies first learn to roll from their stomachs to their backs and from their backs to their stomachs. They raise their heads in stomach lying, then support weight on their elbows, and then their hands. They turn circles on their stomachs and begin to pull themselves forward in an army-crawl fashion. Older babies push up onto their hands and knees to creep. From creeping, they move into and out of sitting. They pull up onto their knees and then stand on their feet. Toddlers begin walking, first with someone holding their hands, and then alone. Preschoolers learn to run, hop, jump, and skip. As you can see, children accomplish many skills in a relatively short period of time.

Individuals with cerebral palsy never experience normal free movement. They are hindered by spasticity or hypotonicity, by abnormal reflexes, and by many other physical, and perhaps mental, problems. Individuals who are severely involved may be unable to perform gross motor skills that babies are capable of.

Physical and occupational therapists work with people who have cerebral palsy to help them learn more normal movements at different developmental levels. Treatment is based on lessening the effects of abnormal reflexes, on facilitating normal balance and postural responses, and on improving the quantity and quality of automatic, voluntary movement. You may see therapists working on rolling, sitting, or stomach lying activities. Individuals with better motor skills can work on creeping and standing. These activities parallel the normal progression of development that was described at the beginning of the chapter. By feeling a normal pattern of movement over and over again during therapy, a person is more likely to be able to copy parts of that movement independently. Treatment is designed to suit each individual's problems and is aimed at increasing functional abilities. For example, the client with spasticity needs to reduce muscle tone, and the client with hemiplegia needs encouragement to use the affected side in a more useful way. These goals can be accomplished through handling techniques, exercise, adaptive equipment, and learning mobility and self-help skills.

The developmental sequence of moving from rolling to hands and knees, to kneeling, to half-kneeling, to standing is an important concept for you to keep in mind in your daily care. The more closely you are able to help the people you care for duplicate these developmental steps in their own movements, the more successful and normal those movements will be. For example, if a client is on the floor and wants to stand, assist the person to hands and knees. Then place a low piece of furniture within reach so the person can push against it to come to kneeling. Help bring one foot forward into a half-kneeling position, and then help the client to stand. The more involved client will need your help to roll in bed and come to a sitting position on the edge in a normal pattern of movement. Pay attention to how you do these movements yourself so you can help the people you work with to do them.

Physical therapists often use bracing devices to correct the alignment of the legs. Spasticity may affect the ankle so that the individual walks on the toes with the foot turned inward. A plastic insert that covers the back of the lower leg, the ankle, and the foot and fits inside the shoe helps to control this tendency. This insert is called an *ankle-foot orthosis* and is made by a specialist called an orthotist. Physical therapists often make similar devices, called splints, that perform similar functions. Not only can splints be made to hold the ankles in position, but they can also be made after surgery to hold the hips, knees, or ankles in positions that aid healing and hold the body part as it was surgically corrected. Metal bracing that is attached to sturdy leather shoes is sometimes used to control the legs. Plastic bracing is usually preferred, however, because the plastic can be specially molded for the individual.

Clients often need assistive devices to help them walk independently. A crutch may have a support that wraps around the lower arm or a support under the armpit. The former type is used most frequently with individuals who have disabilities. Walkers give more help with walking balance than crutches do. Walkers have four legs to provide a large base of support and are pushed along in front of the user. Some have wheels on the front legs for easier pushing. Walkers without wheels have to be lifted slightly with each step, which requires more independent standing balance. If you think one of these devices might help a person you care for, talk to the physical therapist.

You will see physical therapists using many different kinds of equipment with clients. When people with disabilities lose their balance, they often do not know how to shift their weight to regain it, something you do automatically. Physical therapists place clients on large exercise balls, bolsters, and wedges to facilitate more normal balance responses of the upper body and trunk. A large board with a rocker bottom can be used to improve balance reactions in all positions. Clients can sit, crawl, kneel, and stand on a rocker board with assistance and guidance from the therapist. Balance beams and stepladders that lie flat on the floor not only improve balance, but encourage better alignment and strength in walking and teach planning of motor movements.

Chapter 6 illustrated various pieces of positioning equipment and showed how to use them correctly. Remember that it is extremely important for people with disabilities to experience positions that are appropriate for their actual ages. This is one purpose of adaptive equipment. A client who is unable to sit alone can experience sitting in a corner chair or wheelchair. An individual who cannot stand alone can feel what it is like to be upright in a standing frame. Persons with disabilities deserve to be treated with the dignity and respect you would give to a nondisabled person of the same age, and positioning is one aspect of showing this respect.

14
Play and Recreation

Play and recreation are powerful learning tools through which children practice skills and concepts they need to function and participate in life. Through play, we learn how to interact with objects and people in a variety of situations. We learn how to move, manipulate objects, and use our senses. We communicate with others and practice solving problems. By spending enjoyable time in play and recreation, we learn leisure skills we use throughout our adult lives, both with other people and by ourselves.

There are several levels of play. The earliest level is *random* or *exploratory* play, which involves shaking, banging, and exploring the object using different senses. The highest level of play development is *imaginative play,* which is creative, abstract, and imaginative: examples are role playing, and "pretend" play, or "dressing up."

Individuals with disabilities, however, may not be able to play with objects or take part in activities in their surroundings. Because of limited motor movements, they may not be able to turn a knob, wind a toy, or turn on a radio, far less play dress up. Their limited ability to manipulate objects and participate in group activities does not lessen their need to be involved. On the contrary, because of physical limitations, natural opportunities to play may rarely occur. In this section, we will discuss skill development through play and things you as caretakers can do.

Recreation and play develop a variety of skills:

Fine Motor

- To develop reach, grasp, and manipulation skills
- To practice self-help areas, such as self-feeding
- To promote eye-hand coordination

Vision

- To improve visual tracking and scanning
- To increase awareness of the environment

Cognition

- To improve attention to task
- To learn cause-and-effect relationships
- To develop *object permanence* (the understanding that an object continues to exist even when it's out of sight)
- To improve visual and auditory memory

Communication

- To learn that there are things to communicate about and people to communicate with
- To learn language and labeling
- To initiate, maintain, and terminate interactions
- To take turns, in conversation as well as in play

Gross Motor

- To encourage movement
- To practice self-help skills, such as transfers into and out of a chair

One of your many responsibilities in working with people who have special needs is to provide each individual with many different ways to grow and develop as independently as possible. Play or leisure time is an ideal situation for promoting therapy goals, independence, and personal growth of any individual.

Guidelines for Choosing Play and Leisure Activities

1. Know what your goals are in the activity you choose.

   - Is the activity age-appropriate and at the client's cognitive level?
   - Is the activity best enjoyed by the individual alone or by a group?
   - Can the activity be completed independently, or does it require setup or total assistance?
   - Will it be interesting or motivating to the client or group of participants?
   - If the individual cannot manipulate the toys involved, can the game be modified to provide some level of control or participation?

2. Position the client(s) appropriately to reduce the influence of abnormal reflexes and muscle tone. Try alternate positions for play—such as on a wedge, in a corner chair, or sidelying. Reposition the clients, if needed, so they can interact with and touch each other and staff members.

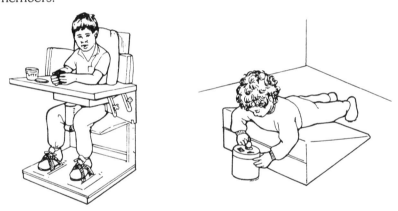

Examples of alternate positions for play

3. Try to make play time as active as possible. Leisure time for people with disabilities is usually passive—for example, watching television or listening to a stereo. When you can allow them active recreation, you have made a significant difference in their lifestyles.

4. Look for ways the person communicates during play. During a more relaxed, leisure activity you often may observe more attempts at interaction or indications of preferences than in a structured program. Signals or communication cues may include these:

   - Looking towards or reaching for a desired object
   - Making eye contact with a peer, staff member, or family member
   - Showing awareness of the presence or absence of an object, person, or action

- Indicating a choice
- Taking turns
- Indicating a desire to continue (or end) an activity

5. Attempt to program peer activities to supplement staff-directed or solitary activities. Staff may, of course, need to set up peer activities, but it can be invaluable for the individuals to control and cooperate during the recreation time. Involving clients in the setup and cleanup also gives them a sense of beginning and ending.

6. Try to allow enough time so the individual or group can participate without feeling rushed. When you are more relaxed, this sense transfers to the clients you are working with and promotes better interactions all around.

7. Most important, enjoy and have fun!

Two frequently asked questions are (1) How do I choose the right toy, game, or activity for a client?, and (2) How do I make an activity age-appropriate for the older client who is at a basic developmental level? In fact, it's not so much a matter of choosing the right toy as using the toy in the right way to address the goal you want to work on. The same toy can be used to encourage communication, fine motor or gross motor skills, or cognition. You can focus on different goals with specific individuals or emphasize several goals simultaneously with the entire group. For example, you could use a tape recorder with a small group for all the following skills:

Listening skills: What was the sound on the tape? Have everyone listen for a certain sound when you play a tape.

Fine motor: Clients select and push control buttons.

Cause-and-effect relationships: Clients can learn that pushing the buttons has the effect of turning the tape recorder on and off.

Turn taking: Structure a game using the tape recorder in which the clients have to use the tape recorder one at a time. Have clients indicate that they want to take a turn in whatever way is appropriate to their skill levels.

Making choices: Clients can choose which tape or song to play.

Positioning: This may be an opportunity to place clients in more upright or functional positions than they are used to—for example, in an upright stander.

Eye contact: Clients can be encouraged to look at the next individual to take a turn, or to staff to end the activity.

Switch use: If the tape player is adapted, clients can practice using switches in a motivating activity.

Choosing age-appropriate toys or activities is often challenging in a group-home setting, where many clients have cognitive skills that are far below their chronological ages. You have to find activities that are appropriate both for the clients' chronological ages and their developmental levels. For example, a baby rattle is never an appropriate choice for an older client who is severely cognitively involved; however, music-based activities, such as playing maracas, a tambourine, or an electronic keyboard, may provide a more age-appropriate way to practice the same skills. Look for activities that are appropriate for any age, such as playing ball, playing musical instruments, or using common household objects, which can give the opportunity to practice basic skills while respecting the individual's chronological age. You can creatively adapt many toys, objects, and games to give your clients enjoyment and a chance to learn and explore.

Glossary of Therapy Terms

abduction: movement out to the sides, away from the middle of the body

access: to gain entry or control of something; for example, *computer access*

activate: to make something happen

active treatment: encouraging the client to participate in formal or informal programming throughout the day, with assistance as needed by staff

adaptive equipment: something that is changed to make its use easier for the client

adduction: movement toward the middle of the body

alignment: arranging or positioning the body in a straight line with the shoulders, hips, knees, and ankles all directly above one another

approximation: pressing two surfaces together

aspiration: taking food or liquid or any foreign substance into the lungs

asymmetry: a difference between two sides of the body; for example, in relative position or muscle tone

ATNR: Asymmetrical tonic neck reflex; an abnormal reflex triggered as the head is turned

augmentative/alternative communication: any system that aids communication by supplementing speech

bird feeding: a position in which the individual is fed with the head and neck tilted back and the mouth open; this is *never* an appropriate position for feeding

cerebral palsy: damage to the brain which happened at or around the time of birth and causes physical or mental disability

cognitive: having to do with thinking skills

communication: the act of sharing information

community-based residence: a homelike setting that provides services to a small group of persons with developmental disabilities

deformities: changes or distortions of the bones or muscles of the body

developmental disability: a severe, chronic mental or physical disability; usually multiple disabilities are present

dislocation: the movement of a bone out of its normal position in a joint

dysfunction: something that is not working or moving correctly

esophagus: the tube that leads from the base of the throat to the stomach; esophageal (adj)

expressive language: the ability to convey a message; for example, by talking, gesturing, pointing

extension: the straightening of a joint or part of the body

external rotation: turning outward of a body part

extremity: a limb such as an arm (upper extremity) or a leg (lower extremity)

facilitate: to make easier or stimulate

fine motor: refers to movements made by the small muscles of the hand, arm, or mouth

flexion: the bending of a body part

fluctuating muscle tone: when the muscle tone in one individual varies from floppy (hypotonic) to stiff (hypertonic)

food texture: the ways in which food or liquid can be presented at a meal, ranging from pureed to regular diet, and from thin to thick liquids

functional: referring to movements that are planned and produce the desired results

gastrostomy (g-tube): feeding through a tube inserted directly into the stomach

gross motor: refers to large muscle movements used to get from one place to another; the muscles used in rolling, crawling, and walking

half-kneeling: a position halfway between kneeling and standing in which the person is on one knee and one foot

hypersensitive: extremely or overly sensitive to some type of sensory input, such as touch

hypertonic/hypertonicity: abnormal stiffness of the muscles; increased (high) muscle tone (see *spasticity*)

hyposensitive: lacking in sensitivity to some type of sensory input, such as touch

hypotonic/hypotonicity: abnormally decreased (low) muscle tone

inhibit: to prevent or decrease

internal rotation: the turning inward of a body part

involuntary: something that happens automatically without thought or effort; something that cannot be consciously controlled, for example, a reflex

joint: the junction between two bones

kyphosis: a curving forward of the spine

language: a symbolic code for expressing thoughts or feelings; one type of communication

midline: an imaginary line down the middle of the body

mobility: the ability to move

motor: the act of moving

multiply handicapped: having more than one disabling problem

muscle tone: the readiness of a muscle to move or support the person

nasogastric tube (NG tube): a tube inserted through the nose directly to the stomach for feeding, not surgically placed

neutral: not favoring either side of the body

non-oral feeding: feeding through any method that is not originated in the mouth

NPO: nothing by mouth, that is, give no food or liquid by mouth

oral motor: movements in or around the mouth

orthosis: a plastic splint or brace that is specially molded for an individual to help protect, support, or correct the position of a body part or to assist with a particular function, such as holding a pencil

palate: the roof of the mouth

passive movement: movement without voluntary effort on the part of the client

passive range of motion: taking a limb through all the positions it can move to without participation from the individual

pathology: the study of changes produced by disease; a change produced by disease

perception: taking in information through the senses and acting on it

pharynx: the back of the throat

pivot transfer: moving from one place to another by turning the body

plaque: gummy film containing bacteria that builds up on the enamel of teeth

positioning: a way of being placed

radial: toward the thumb side of the hand

range of motion: the direction and amount of movement a joint is capable of

receptive language: the language you are able to understand

reciprocal: refers to an alternating movement or action; for example, one leg up and one leg down

reflexes: an involuntary response to a touch, sound, movement, or change of position

reflux: backwards flow of the stomach contents into the esophagus

retracted: pulled back; for example, shoulders or lips may be retracted by increased muscle tone

rotation: twisting of a body part in a circular direction; for example, the shoulders turning to the left while the hips remain stationary

scoliosis: a sideways curve of the spine

sensation: an awareness of feeling or of being able to feel

spastic diplegia: a type of cerebral palsy that affects mainly the legs

spastic hemiplegia: a type of cerebral palsy that affects one side of the body

spasticity: high muscle tone causing stiff and awkward movements (see *hypertonic*)

spastic quadriplegia: a type of cerebral palsy that affects the entire body

speech: sounds produced by the mouth that are used in language (as distinct from *vegetative* sounds, such as coughing)

stabilizing: holding steady

stereotyped: repetitive behavior, happening over and over

stimulate: to arouse

suckling: a backward and forward movement of the tongue that moves food back in the mouth for swallowing

switch mechanism: a device to control an object or something in the environment

symmetry: both sides of the body look the same

tactile defensiveness: a heightened response to touch

transfer: moving from one place to another

Appendix: Equipment Sources

These lists do not imply recommendations of any company. We recommend comparative pricing.

Adaptive Equipment: General

Alimed, Inc.
297 High Street
Dedham, MA 02026
800-225-2610

Cleo, Inc.
3957 Mayfield Road
Cleveland, OH 44121
800-321-0595

Fred Sammons, Inc.
Box 32
Brookfield, IL 60513-0032
800-323-5547

G. E. Miller
484 S. Broadway
P.O. Box 266
Yonkers, NY 10705
800-431-2924

Heartland
P.O. Box 1151
Sterling, IL 61081
800-225-9489

J. A. Preston
60 Page Road
Clifton, NJ 07012
800-631-7277

Maddak, Inc.
Pequannock, NJ 07440-1993
201-694-0500

North Coast Medical, Inc.
450 Salmar Ave.
Campbell, CA 95008
800-821-9319

Smith and Nephew Rolyan, Inc.
N93 W14475 Whittaker Way
Menomonee Falls, WI 53051
800-558-8633

Southside Apothecary
1351 Mt. Hope Ave.
Rochester, NY 14620
716-217-7141

Positioning Equipment

Achievement Products
P.O. Box 547
Mineola, NY 11501
516-747-8899

Alimed, Inc.
297 High Street
Dedham, MA 02026
800-225-2610

Best Priced Products, Inc.
P.O. Box 1174
White Plains, NY 10602
800-824-2934

Cleo, Inc.
3957 Mayfield Road
Cleveland, OH 44121
800-321-0595

Danmar Products, Inc.
2390 Winewood
Ann Arbor, MI 48103
313-761-1990

Equipment Shop
P.O. Box 33
Bedford, MA 01730
617-275-7681

Flaghouse, Inc.: Special
Populations
150 N. MacQuesten Parkway
Mt. Vernon, NY 10550
800-221-5185

Fred Sammons, Inc.
Box 32
Brookfield, IL 60513-0032
800-323-5547

J. A. Preston
60 Page Road
Clifton, NJ 07012
800-631-7277

Jesana, Ltd.
P.O. Box 17
Irvington, NY 10533
800-443-4728

Kaye Products, Inc.
1010 E. Pettigrew St.
Durham, NC 27701-4299
919-732-6444

Maddak, Inc.
Pequannock, NJ 07440-1993
201-694-0500

Motor Development Corporation
P.O. Box 4054
Downey, CA 90241
213-862-6741

North Coast Medical, Inc.
450 Salmar Ave.
Campbell, CA 95008
800-821-9319

Pen Dot Products
8100 Austin Avenue
Morton Grove, IL 60053-9801
312-470-7885

Rifton
Route 213
Rifton, NY 12471
914-658-3141

Southpaw Enterprises, Inc.
800 W. Third Street
Dayton, OH 45407-2805
800-228-1698

Therapy Skill Builders
3830 E. Bellevue
P.O. Box 42050
Tucson, AZ 85733
602-323-7500

Play Equipment/
Educational Materials

Achievement Products
P.O. Box 547
Mineola, NY 11501
516-747-8899

The Capable Child
8 Herkiner Ave.
Hewlett, NY 11557
516-872-1603

Chime Time
934 Anderson Drive
Homer, NY 13077
800-423-KIDS

Community Playthings
Route 213
Rifton, NY 12471
914-658-3141

Danmar Products, Inc.
2390 Winewood
Ann Arbor, MI 48103
313-761-1990

DLM Teaching Resources
P.O. Box 4000
One DLM Park
Allen, TX 75002
800-527-4747

Equipment Shop
P.O. Box 33
Bedford, MA 01730
617-275-7681

Flaghouse, Inc.: Special
Populations
150 N. MacQuesten Parkway
Mt. Vernon, NY 10550
800-221-5185

J. A. Preston
60 Page Road
Clifton, NJ 07012
800-631-7277

Jesana, Ltd.
P.O. Box 17
Irvington, NY 10533
800-443-4728

Kapable Kids
P.O. Box 250
Bohemia, NY 11716
516-563-7176

Kaye Products, Inc.
1010 E. Pettigrew St.
Durham, NC 27701-4299
919-732-6444

Kids and Things
Pequannock, NJ 07440-1993
201-694-0500

The Preschool Source
6500 Peachtree Ind. Blvd.
P.O. Box 4750
Norcross, GA 30091
800-247-6623

Salco Toys, Inc.
11445 150th St. E.
Nerstrand, MN 55053

Southpaw Enterprises, Inc.
800 W. Third Street
Dayton, OH 45407-2805
800-228-1698

Switch Mechanisms/ Augmentative Communication

Ablenet
1081 10th Avenue S.E.
Minneapolis, MN 55414
612-379-0956

Adaptive Communication
Systems, Inc.
P.O. Box 12440
Pittsburgh, PA 15231
412-264-2288

Adaptive Peripherals, Inc.
4529 Bagley Ave. North
Seattle, WA 98103
206-633-2610

The Capable Child
8 Herkiner Ave.
Hewlett, NY 11557
516-872-1603

Canon USA, Inc.
One Canon Plaza
Lake Success, NY 11042
516-488-6700

Creative Switch Industries
P.O. Box 5256
Des Moines, IA 50306
515-287-5748

Developmental Equipment, Inc.
P.O. Box 639
1000 N. Rand Road,
Building 115
Wauconda, IL 60084
312-526-2682

DLM Teaching Resources
P.O. Box 4000
One DLM Park
Allen, TX 75002
800-527-4747

Flaghouse, Inc.: Special
Populations
150 N. MacQuesten Parkway
Mt. Vernon, NY 10550
800-221-5185

Jesana, Ltd.
P.O. Box 17
Irvington, NY 10533
800-443-4728

Kapable Kids
P.O. Box 250
Bohemia, NY 11716
516-563-7176

Loqui Systems
Suite 109-327
15466 Los Gatos Blvd.
Los Gatos, CA 95032
408-356-7256

Maddak, Inc.
Pequannock, NJ 07440-1993
210-694-0500

Medical Technology Systems, Inc.
90 Great Oaks Blvd.
San Jose, CA 95119
408-224-6324

Phonic Ear, Inc.
250 Camino Alto
Mill Valley, CA 94941
415-383-4000

Prentke Romich Company
1022 Heyl Road
Wooster, OH 44691
216-262-1984

Salco Toys, Inc.
11445 150th St. E.
Nerstrand, MN 55053

Sentient Systems Technology, Inc.
5001 Baum Blvd.
Pittsburgh, PA 15213
412-682-0144

Sonoma State Hospital/
Development Center
Communication Engineering
P.O. Box 1493
Eldridge, CA 95431
707-938-6306

Steven Kamor, Ph.D., Inc.
8 Main Street
Hastings-on-Hudson, NY 10706
914-478-0960

Tash
70 Gibson Drive, Unit 12
Markham, Ontario, Canada L3R
4C2
416-475-2212

Therapy Skill Builders
3830 E. Bellevue
P.O. Box 42050
Tucson, AZ 85733
602-323-7500

Unicorn Engineering Company
6201 Harwood Ave.
Oakland, CA 94618
415-428-1626

Wayne County Intermediate
School District
3350 Van Born Road
Wayne, MI 48184

Zygo Industries, Inc.
P.O. Box 1008
Portland, OR 97207-1008
503-297-1424

Adaptive Equipment:
Feeding and Oral-Motor

A-Plus Products
P.O. Box 2975
Beverly Hills, CA 90213

Achievement Products
P.O. Box 547
Mineola, NY 11501
516-747-8899

Ansa Bottle Company, Inc.
1107 W. Shawnee
Muskogee, OK 74401

Baby World Company, Inc.
Station Plaza East
Great Neck, NY 11021

Cleo, Inc.
3957 Mayfield Road
Cleveland, OH 44121
800-321-0595

Current, Inc.
The Current Building
Colorado Springs, CO 80941

Cutoy Cooperative Association
P.O. Box 22057
Los Angeles, CA 90022

Equipment Shop
P.O. Box 33
Bedford, MA 01730
617-275-7681

Evenflo Products Company
771 N. Freedom Street
Ravenna, OH 44266

The First Years
1 Kiddy Drive
Avon, MA 02322

Fred Sammons, Inc.
Box 32
Brookfield, IL 60513-0032
800-323-5547

Gerber Products Company
445 State Street
Fremont, MI 49412

Gus File, Inc.
Albuquerque, NM 87110

Happy Baby, Inc.
P.O. Box 557
Crystal Lake, IL 60014

Heartland
P.O. Box 1151
Sterling, IL 61081
800-225-9489

H. J. Heinz Company
Pittsburgh, PA 15212

Infa, Inc.
3301 W. Meade Ave.
Las Vegas, NV 89102

International Associates, Inc.
P.O. Box 87321
Atlanta, GA 30337

J. A. Preston
60 Page Road
Clifton, NJ 07012
800-631-7277

Johnson and Johnson Baby
Products Company
Skillman, NJ 08558

Just for Kids Catalog
Winterbrook Way
Meredith, NH 03253

Kaye's Kids Catalog
1010 E. Pettigrew St.
Durham, NC 27701-4299
919-732-6444

Lact-Aid International, Inc.
P.O. Box 10-66
Athens, TN 37303

Lakeshore Curriculum Materials
2695 E. Dominguez Street/P.O.
Box 1209
Carson, CA 90749

Maddak, Inc.
Pequannock, NJ 07440-1993
201-694-0500

Marriott Concepts
Box 1335
Orem, UT 84057

Marshall Baby Care Products
Division of Marshall Electronics,
Inc.
600 Barclay Blvd.
Lincolnshire, IL 60065

Mead Johnson Company
Nutritional Division
Evansville, IN 47721

Medeal
P.O. Box 386
Crystal Lake, IL 60014

North Coast Medical, Inc.
450 Salmar Ave.
Campbell, CA 95008
800-821-9319

Playskool, Inc.
108 Fairway Court
Northvale, NJ 07647

Playtex
P.O. Box 728
Paramus, NJ 07652

Quanterron, Inc.
11531 Rupp Drive
Burnsville, MN 55378

Sanitoy, Inc.
1 Nursery Lane
Fitchburg, MA 01420

Sassy, Inc.
191 Waukegan Road
Northfield, IL 60093

Small World Toys
P.O. Box 5291
Beverly Hills, CA 90210

Smith and Nephew Rolyan, Inc.
N93 W14475 Whittaker Way
Menomonee Falls, WI 53051
800-558-8633

Solo Cup Company
1505 E. Main
Urbana, IL 61801

Stanmar Manufacturing Co.
131 Brokaw Road
San Jose, CA 95112

Therapy Skill Builders
3830 E. Bellevue
P.O. Box 42050
Tucson, AZ 85733
602-323-7500

Tommee Tippee
Playskool, Inc.
108 Fairway Court
Northvale, NJ 07647

Tupperware Home Products
P.O. Box 2353
Orlando, FL 32802
800-858-7221

Bibliography

Bobath, B. 1985. *Abnormal postural reflex activity caused by brain lesions.* Rockville, MD: Aspen Systems Corporation.

Bruner, J. S. 1973. *The power of play.* Garden City, NY: Anchor Press.

Conner, F. P., G. G. Williamson, and J. M. Siepp. 1978. *Program guide for infants and toddlers with neuromotor and other developmental disabilities.* New York: Teachers College Press.

Costello, J. M., and A. L. Holland. 1986. *Handbook of speech and language disorders.* San Diego, CA: College-Hill Press.

Davis, H., and S. R. Silverman. 1978. *Hearing and deafness.* New York: Holt, Rinehart, and Winston.

Finnie, N. 1975. *Handling the young cerebral palsied child at home.* New York: Dutton and Co.

Harrell, L., and N. Akeson. 1987. *Preschool vision stimulation: It's more than a flashlight.* New York: American Foundation for the Blind.

Kenny, D. J., and P. L. Judd. 1988. Oral care for developmentally disabled children: The primary dentition stage. *Infants and Young Children* 1(2):11-19.

King, M. L. 1984. *Parenting preschoolers: Suggestions for raising young blind and visually impaired children.* New York: American Foundation for the Blind.

Logeman, J. A. 1986. *Manual for the videofluorographic study of swallowing.* San Diego, CA: College-Hill Press.

Morris, S. E., and M. K. Dunn. 1987. *Pre-feeding skills.* Tucson, AZ: Therapy Skill Builders.

Musselwhite, C. R., and K. W. St. Louis. 1982. *Communication programming for the severely handicapped: Vocal and non-vocal strategies.* San Diego, CA: College-Hill Press.

Northern, J. L. 1976. *Hearing disorders.* Boston: Little, Brown and Company.

Seiler, C. 1988. Sweet medicines tough on teeth? *Wheat Ridge Regional Center Bulletin.* Wheat Ridge, CO: Wheat Ridge Regional Center.